# Dusting off the Ashes
## One Man's Personal Journey Through Post-Traumatic Stress

Maria Heaton, M.S.
as told by William Curtin

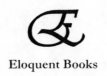

Eloquent Books

Eloquent Books
An imprint of Strategic Book Group
P.O. Box 333
Durham CT 06422
www.StrategicBookGroup.com

ISBN: 978-1-60860-925-3

Printed in the United States of America

Book Design: Stacie Tingen

*To John, Giavanna, and Jacob,*
*Thank you for everything, especially your encouragement*

For the memory of my dear friends who perished on September 11, 2001. This book was inspired for you and for all others who survived, but whose lives were altered forever.


You will always be in my heart,
Bill

# Introduction

Many people do not know how to acknowledge post-traumatic stress disorder (PTSD). This applies to both society in general and the victims themselves. Men and women returning from war, victims of abuse, and survivors of other horrific, life-changing events often are not supported by society with the follow-up treatment that they so desperately need. In so many cases, they are left twisting in the wind and their lives are never the same.

When William Curtin Jr. came to my office and told his story, I found myself wondering how he seemingly managed to be doing so well. I was surprised by his outgoing personality and pleasant façade, only to find that life for him was difficult at best. At that time, Bill had been to two different therapists and had simply resigned himself to a life that was very different from the way he had lived for the previous twenty-four years. When I met him, Bill was living in Bethlehem, Pennsylvania in a small one-bedroom apartment. His only income was Social Security disability. Together we worked through his depression as I assisted Bill in finding new direction in his life and reconnecting with his children. Some time after our counseling had ceased, he showed me a brown journal that he had used to write down his thoughts and feelings. He asked me to take it home to read. Bill expressed an interest in putting his life, mainly his experience on September 11th, onto paper. "I want to tell my story," he once told me, "but I'm not very good at writing." He asked me for help, and together we created this book.

This memoir's pivotal moment occurs when Bill finds himself in the middle of the September 11 tragedy, which ultimately leads him to seek therapy and to confront situations going on at home. Bill's story is so much more than 9/11: living with an alcoholic, abusive father, "parenting" his siblings and playing the "husband" to his mother, the 1993 World Trade Center bombing, his wife's addiction to prescription drugs, and the ultimate destruction of his family. At times, the book is difficult to read because of its graphic details, and yet you cannot stop reading because you want to know what happens next. Woven throughout is Bill's uplifting sense of faith and belief.

This book contains many grotesque details which I was at first hesitant to include. However, the events of September 11 did happen, and this book would serve no purpose if it did not describe the events as Bill experienced them. The gory details are not intended to entertain; instead, they are a vehicle to help those who have suffered, either as a result of 9/11 or from another trauma. Victims of war, abuse, severe loss, or other tragedies, as well as survivors and loved ones, have all experienced many of the emotions described here. Those who are still walking around in their own state of shock and disbelief may find comfort in knowing that they are not alone.

Many people died on that horrible day we now refer to only as 9/11, but many others also stopped living. The survivors who escaped unscathed physically all share a death that will stay with them forever. For those who were there, it was as if they had been sent to war without the proper training. They found themselves in a situation where they had to meet death head on. Some joined together to comfort one another; others walked away in sheer disbelief only to realize that, although they may have survived, they are suffering from an affliction called post-traumatic stress disorder. Survivors may be you or I, functioning in the world today but with nightmares, emptiness, and fear. While post-traumatic stress may paralyze an individual, it also causes a person to re-live the tragic events repeatedly in their mind.

This book is first an affirmation to all of you who have been there and survived. To you, I applaud your strength and wish you the peacefulness you so deserve. It is also a book of hope, written to show you that there is help for you and that you may be able to live life again and begin to feel as you once did.

Through the eyes of darkness let there be light
In times of tragedy let there be hope
When your last piece of sanity feels like it is slipping from
your grasp
Find comfort that you are not alone and hold onto it today as
tightly as you can
Because tomorrow holds a new peacefulness
That will embrace you and allow you to carry on.

-Maria Heaton-

# Table of Contents

# *Acknowledgments*

When Bill Curtin first asked me if I would like to write a book about his life, I was very excited. I soon realized, however, that it was not going to be an easy task. Trying to summarize the events of a person's life within a number of pages is difficult at best. However, after working with Bill on almost a daily basis, he began to tell his story in such a manner that I felt I was living it with him. His complete and total cooperation and willingness to expose his innermost feelings and personal moments will always be appreciated. I thank him for that and for allowing me the freedom to tell his story in the manner in which it is written. Many times, it was not easy for him to recall certain events without becoming emotional, but Bill continued to work with me, as he felt it his purpose to share with others so that they may be able to overcome and find hope.

Several other people have helped me in my career these past years, one of whom is Frances Gaal, Ph.D. As I went back for an advanced degree to pursue a career in counseling, Dr. Gaal served as my mentor and my friend. Without his guidance, knowledge, and support, I would not have been able to do the work that I do in private practice today. I would also like to thank Geta Vogel, Ed.Sp., who mentored and supervised me throughout my many years at the Warren County Technical School. Geta supported me and taught me the finer points of educational counseling and helping individuals succeed in life. Christine Blackston provided assistance with all of the editing for this book. Many nights I sat with her and read each chapter, each sentence, to make sure the reader would fully grasp the emotions that I was trying to convey. Kristen Depken was a tremendous help in reading and editing the final drafts. Lastly, I would like to thank my husband and two children for their support and patience whenever I needed help, feedback or just an occasional ear to bounce ideas off of. Their kind words of encouragement are not forgotten.

## Chapter One

# *My Childhood in New York City*

The minute I felt the rumble and heard the loud explosion, I knew something was very, very wrong. My instincts told me to get out of the building and run. I did just that. I grabbed my jacket and wallet, said goodbye to my coworkers, and with much trepidation made my way to the street below. When I got outside it seemed as if everyone had disappeared. I looked up and saw a huge, gaping hole in the side of the North Tower. The street was very quiet. It felt like I was the only one there. I gazed back up at the tower again in disbelief, only to see the same gigantic hole that cut into the side of the building. Papers were raining down and small flames stretched out from where the plane had entered. I could see the defined outline of a jet-liner, where the aircraft had penetrated the side of the building. *There's no way that was a Cessna,* I thought to myself. There was a distinctive smell of jet fuel in the air. Confusion came over me. I was dazed. I looked over to the area where I purchased my coffee each day and noticed an empty cart. No one was on the street. I was all alone. I had no idea, looking up at the tower at that point, how many people were already dead.

I stood there for what seemed like minutes but was probably only seconds. I am sure I was in shock at that moment. I was startled awake by the sound of sirens heading toward me as I became aware of others running in panic. I decided to go left, up Park Place to West Broadway. When I reached that corner, I turned right and started walking toward the South Tower. I crossed the street there because I was not able to see the North Tower from that position and I wanted to get out of the way of the people who were now emerging from the buildings and coming toward me. My decision to cross the street saved my life that day. As I got closer to the towers, I stopped and realized people were crying. One woman was vomiting, saying, "People are jumping." *Of course, people don't jump, she must be crazy*, I thought to myself. Then I looked up at the sky again. The smoke was thicker and the flames around the tower had grown more intense. What I saw next was the most unimaginable event I have ever witnessed.

As I sit here today, July 5, 2005, my 48th birthday, and begin to write, I realize so many things have happened to me in my life. I feel very lost in my mind. The loss of my family, friends, and all the other special people who have helped to mold me over the course of my life, both spiritually and morally, can make it hard for me to do something as natural as breathing at times. I often think of how I imagined my life would be. You know those pictures we have in our heads? We develop those pictures and form our own personal photo album from the day we start to dream about how we see ourselves in the world. After living life so far, I have come to realize that none of us really controls anything in our lives and, because of that, the pictures in our photo albums must change. Some photos we do not mind discarding. It is the others, the ones that remain in our minds and our hearts and that we cannot let go of, that can make our journey ever so difficult. The death of my friends on September 11 and, eventually, the end of my twenty-five year marriage and prosperous career

4

have forced me to look at my album and make changes in order for me to survive and allow myself to be happy again.

As I tell my story, I continue to wonder whether the decisions I have made throughout my life were correct or were too influenced by the severe traumas bestowed upon me. I believe that when you suffer such trauma in your life, you begin to feel lost. Although everyone is trying to help, you just feel more lost with each passing moment. I have found that whomever I spoke to always gave me their perspective on what they would have done. I cannot help but think that, if they were in my shoes, they would probably crumble. Death has tried to pay me a visit several times in my life. The question that has been with me for many years and remains unanswered today is *Why? Why has my life been spared?* The horrific memories replay in my mind almost every day. Sometimes I think I may know why; other times I simply must trust that God has a bigger plan lined up for me, one I have not yet seen. Perhaps with the writing of this book, someone who may need my assistance will cross my path one day. Whatever the reason, I hope that by sharing my experiences I can help others who are still suffering in silence.

These past years were spent in many therapy sessions trying to comprehend what happened on 9/11. My experience was terrible and the worst thing that I ever encountered in my life. Here is my story.

\*\*\*

My normal day began at 4:30 a.m. as it had for the previous twenty-four years. Between the demands of work and the desire to be a good husband and father, it was very stressful for me. I worked on Wall Street as a money market broker, which carried its own amount of stress.

After many counseling sessions, I now realize that I had been on the verge of a nervous breakdown but refused to stop what I was doing because I had no safety net upon which to fall. I was the main breadwinner. I was where it started and ended. There were many mornings when it was freezing or snowing so hard I could not believe I had to go out in it, but Wall Street does not care about weather conditions. "You need to be here" was the mantra. When you build up a client base, the clients only want to deal with you. No one else will do.

I had worked my way up as a runner on the street delivering stock certificates. With only a high school education and not much else, I was determined not to become my father. He had been an abusive alcoholic my entire life. He was also a broker in New York; however, that is where our similarities ended. My father often beat me for seemingly no reason; but when I think back, it began when my mom started working at night to move us out of New York City. That is where I was born—the Bronx to be exact.

My mother went to work as a telephone operator from 6:00 p.m. until 1:00 a.m. each night. My younger sister Connie and I would come home from school and play outside for a couple hours until my mom had to go to work. Mom would stick her head out the window and yell, "Get your asses up here!" That is how my mother would talk. She did not really curse, but when she was mad, you knew it.

Because she would be out all evening and there were three kids home at the time, my mom expected my dad to come home after work, get dinner and take care of us. He failed at this, mostly because his primary loyalty was to the corner tavern. Therefore, at the age of nine, the job fell to me to care for my two sisters, ages six and one. We lived in a two-bedroom apartment on the third floor. I would change my baby sister Marie's diapers and prepare our dinners. Pampers were not an option back then; I used real diapers with real safety pins, a huge responsibility for a nine-year-old. My mom taught me how to lift my youngest sister out of the crib, holding the back of her neck carefully so as not to let her head flip back. After changing her diaper, I would heat up her bottle in a pot on the stove. She would take her bottle and I would burp her before I got dinner ready for Connie and me. Then we would play with Marie until bedtime. I was the only son and the oldest child. My father was very unreliable when it came to his family so the responsibility always fell to me, taking care of things around the house for my mom.

I would get scared when it got dark because I knew that the roaches would be coming out. Once we were asleep, they would actually crawl into our beds. I could not believe we had to live this way, and I often wondered if other kids also had to live like this. To keep from falling asleep, Connie and I would make up games and play until our dad came home. Drunk. Always drunk. I did not really understand the concept of time at that age. All I knew was that it was dark. We would watch TV in my parent's room until I heard my father's key opening the lock in the front door. If I had dozed off, I would jump up in their bed so he would not yell at me for being asleep while I was supposed to be watching my sisters. He would always go straight into the kitchen looking for food, cursing and mumbling under

7

his breath about how shitty his life was. "Fuckin' kids. I got no life. There's no dinner, she's not home, and she's out working." It was a dual conversation with a solo performer and neither party won. He was pissed off at the world and we all knew it, but we were not quite sure why. He continued this jargon as he stumbled to his bed and fell asleep, in most cases with a lit cigarette.

Later, when my mom would call, I would tell her he had gotten home late, and she would ask to speak to him. When they finished their conversation, I would get a beating for telling my mom that my dad had just gotten home. This went on all through my younger years, night after night. I never remember a moment at home where I could just relax and be a kid. The responsibility was overwhelming, yet it was common for me to function this way. I did not realize these were not normal circumstances for a boy my age because nobody talked about it.

I have an unusual ability to bring back crystal-clear pictures of my childhood memories (as well as the rest of my life). It is almost like being able to recall them by pressing play or rewind buttons on a VCR that has a library of all my home movies.

Some of my fondest memories include my grandmother, known to me as Nanny. She and my grandfather were Irish immigrants who landed on Ellis Island in 1930 and settled in the Bronx. They were my mom's parents. I never knew my grandfather because he died of a heart attack at the age of forty-three, when my mother was a young teenager. In my memory, Nan was forever mourning his death. When my grandfather died, they had three children: my mom, Aunt Flo and Uncle John. Thirteen when I was born, Uncle John became like a brother to me. My Nan lived in a small one-bedroom, walk-in apartment one block from where my parents lived. I attended Catholic grade school, St. Simon Stock, and proudly wore my Catholic school uniform with my necktie (dark blue with yellow embroidery, S.S.S.). We were given an hour-and-fifteen-minute break from classes each day, and I would walk over to my Nan's for lunch. Every day she waited at her door with a quarter for me so that I could go to the corner store to buy my favorite snack, Dipsy Doodles. When I got back, she would sit me on her footstool and feed me a soft-boiled egg. The coup de grace was the plate of bacon and sausage afterwards. Yes, I truly was a young Irish prince in her eyes. We would talk, and I spent many nights sleeping over on the weekends. I felt so safe and secure, knowing that I would not be dealing with the fighting, yelling and physical abuse that went on at my house. I pray to Nanny every day, and I have never forgotten the overwhelming impact she had on my life.

My first near-death experience occurred when I was eight years old. I had just gotten a brand-new bike for my birthday from my Uncle John. It was the most beautiful bicycle I had ever seen in my life. It had a banana seat with "V" handlebars and knobby tires. The color was metallic silver with maroon stripes. It was awesome.

It was a normal day like any other, and I could not wait to get out and ride my new bike around the neighborhood. My uncle had told me not to take it out without him, but I could not wait. I convinced my Nan to let me ride up to the corner tavern and back. When my feet hit the pedals, it was magic. It was a cool bike and, in my head, I imagined everyone watching me in envy, all wanting to have one. It had started to rain, and

I was going to take one more spin around the block. I did not even get to the end of my street when a kid jumped out from between two parked cars, put a gun to my head and told me to get off the bike. There were only two choices for me at that moment: ride away and risk getting shot or surrender my new prized possession. I handed over the bike without a fight. As I watched the kid pedal away with my new bike, I stood frozen in shock with tears streaming down my face. Although I had lost my bike, I was very lucky that he had not pulled the trigger, and I never forgot it.

From that day on, I was very aware of my surroundings. Every person around me was suspect and I became sensitive to people's movements. I transitioned from an eight-year-old boy to an eight-year-old man emotionally. The innocence was gone. That was the first time death tried to pay me a visit. That incident was the major reason my mom decided it was time to get out of the city. She knew our neighborhood was in slow decay and was not going to get any better. That is when she started working more at night to save money so that we could leave New York. That is also when the real beatings began.

Dangerous situations continued to come and go in my life. When I was nine years old, I went down to the second floor of our apartment building to visit my Aunt Flo. I stupidly left the door to my aunt's apartment ajar and went into the back bedroom where my aunt was on the telephone. Shortly after, we heard someone banging around in the kitchen. She asked me, "Billy, did you lock the door?" She then screamed, prompting me to run behind the bedroom door. I was shaking and thinking that whoever was in her apartment would come in and kill us both. My aunt screamed down the hall to the darkness: "I'm calling the cops!" I guess the intruder left at that point because we heard footsteps running toward the front door. My aunt called my mom, and she came running down the stairs with a huge kitchen knife in her hand. She yelled for us to come out and, fortunately, whoever was there had already gone. My mom opened up the closet and started stabbing the clothes inside, thinking the intruder was still in there hiding.

I never forgot that fear. In fact, after that incident, when my mom went to work and my dad did not come home at night, I used to urinate in a cup in the kitchen and pour it down the sink. The bathroom was on the other side of the apartment, in the dark, and I was always afraid someone was in there hiding, waiting to get me.

Every Sunday, my mother would take us to Mass. All of my relatives were of a strict Irish-Catholic persuasion, so we attended Mass every Sunday. I was even an altar boy for three years. Little did I know how my faith in God would carry me through many difficult times in my life. I feel that many guardian angels have kept a constant watch over me.

We went to Catholic school at the time, and you had to be in line and enter the church with your class for Mass. You had to be there. If you were not, you had to have a good reason. After Mass, we would usually stop at the bakery on our walk home. One day, my mom ran into some of her friends on the way out of church and starting talking. She wore a huge flowery hat and, as we stood waiting, she said, "Billy, do me a favor. Run down to the bakery and buy me a half dozen seeded rolls." I agreed, and so she gave me some money and said, "Get right back. I'll be waiting here." Halfway down the block, I noticed my friends in an abandoned car on the corner, jumping in and out and yelling for me to come join them. Of course, I jumped in even though I was wearing my church suit, and we started fooling around until a man came out of a nearby building and yelled at us to get off the car. I looked at him and gave a rude hand gesture, and he came after me. I jumped out of the car and ran around the corner into the basement of an abandoned apartment building.

Now, all this time my mom was still chatting away on the corner, thinking that I was at the bakery getting her rolls. Even though I was only nine years old, I felt like I was twenty because I already knew a lot about the streets. Two of my friends and I took off in one direction while our three other friends went the other way, thinking the man couldn't follow all of us. But he came after my friends and I. We went into an alley feeling safe, as if we had really gotten something over on this guy, when all of a sudden I saw an arm with a large hand grab my buddy by the nape of the neck and snap him back. "I'll kick your asses," said the man. I frantically took off, left the man and my friends there, and went to the bakery to get my mom's rolls. After purchasing the rolls, my two friends had regrouped outside the bakery after their escape from him, and were waiting for me to come out. We decided to go around the block, taking the long way back to my mother in an effort to avoid the man who was still looking for us. We passed a woman who was sweeping the sidewalk outside her apartment. Obviously not getting our fill of trouble, my friends and I yelled something to her, a smart-ass remark with a hand gesture. To our surprise, her husband pulled up behind us in his car and yelled, "What'd you say to her?" With that, he grabbed *me* by the back of the neck and said, "I heard what you said to her! Why did you say that?" He grabbed my friend, too. I started to cry because he held me so hard. The woman then yelled for him to leave us alone, and he let go, adding, "If I ever see you fuckin' guys here again I'll put that fuckin' broom up your ass." That is how people talked where we came from.

When I finally got back to my mom, she asked where I had been and why my face was so flushed. Being the pale Irish red-head, you could see the red mark on the back of my neck. I told her a man had just grabbed me. "I'm gonna go talk to that guy," she said angrily, but I told her to leave it alone. She insisted on telling my father, however, and as we walked up the steps, I was certain that he was going to beat the heck out of me. I felt like I was going to soil my trousers. But, despite all the times he had beaten me for no reason, this time he called me into the room and said, "I'm only gonna ask you one time. What happened? And I am warning you, don't lie to me. Don't let me go down there and ask that guy if you did something wrong." I told him in a low tone, almost under my breath, what I had said to the lady. "Okay," my father said. "Go to your room. Don't come out for the rest of the day." No beatings, nothing. I was in shock. That is when I realized that I would get in less trouble for telling the truth. That was a defining moment for me. I looked at him and understood what he meant for the first time when he told me, "You have to be able to tell someone the truth because then they can help you." I realized that you could trust someone and say, "This is what I did," and move on, and at least your soul would be cleansed. You do not have to tell five versions of the same story. This has been my philosophy ever since.

Living in New York was rough. My parents had no idea how terrible it was for me. When I was in elementary school, the older gang of kids made us snort bags of airplane glue in order to get into our apartment building after school. If we refused, they would beat us up. The Negroes often spit on my friends and me when we were walking home from school. They would wait for us to cross Grand Concourse. We had to fight every day just to survive. I knew the black and white thing was wrong, and I did not understand the whole hate thing. I just needed to get home each day and knew they had a problem with my skin color.

The first black student we ever had in class was in the third grade. His name was Julius. I helped him after school when the white kids were beating him up. I tried to stop them from hurting him at the expense of getting the shit kicked out of me. He was so grateful that he waited outside my apartment building and wanted to carry my books to school. It felt good to help him. Luckily for me, I had not inherited the hatred my father had burning so deeply inside of him. Even at that young age, I was ferociously determined not to become like *him*.

By the spring of 1969, when I was twelve, my mom had saved up enough money for a down payment on a new house, and my father got a job as the head teller at the Ramapo Bank in Lakeland, New Jersey. My parents announced to the rest of the family their decision to move. My Nan would often sit me on her lap at night and sing "ole" Irish songs. She would finish with a kiss on the back of my head, telling me she loved me very much. She was extremely heartbroken that I would be leaving soon but happy that we were going to be getting out of the city. Soon after we moved away, she got very sick and asked my mom to send my sister Connie and me to come visit her. I went first and spent a week. My sister went the following week. Nan passed away in her sleep while Connie was there. This was something my sister never forgot. It almost seemed like my Nan made sure that we were safe and finally out of New York City and then was able to let go. Many of my mannerisms come from her, as do my respect for elderly people, my way of speaking to adults, and, most of all, my belief in God. I will always remember that short, very frail, gray-haired woman in a day dress with a long-sleeved sweater, her hair pulled back into a bun with bobby pins and her nylon stockings rolled up to her kneecaps. She stays forever in my mind, waiting for me to come home to her apartment for my lunch.

# Chapter Two

## *Growing Up*

When we moved out of New York, I was in the start of my sixth-grade year. Our new home was a very different place in both location and environment. Vernon Valley, New Jersey was a long way up from where we had come. I mean way up. Cows and farms surrounded us, a completely new environment. It was a total change from the way I had been used to living. By now my mom had given birth to my third sister, Lynne. My father took the one car we had to work each day so my mother, my sisters and I had no way to get anywhere. It was okay though, as the isolation brought us very close to each other.

I wore a suit to my first day at my new school because that is what I was accustomed to wearing in Catholic school. It was my first day ever in a public school environment. When I got there, every other kid was in jeans and a t-shirt. I looked like a real ass and all the kids let me know it. They treated me as if I had the plague. It was difficult starting there; nobody wanted to talk to me and it took weeks before anyone accepted me, which was purely by accident. During a football game in gym class, another student fumbled a pass and I grabbed it right out of the air and ran a touchdown. Everyone was clapping and I felt like a big hero. I quickly realized that sports were an avenue to instant acceptance when you were good at them.

Over the next few years I made a few friends and was able to fit into a more laid-back country setting. Meanwhile, things at home continued to get progressively worse. My dad was an angry man. His home life as a child had been one of alcoholism and abuse. His parents had come over from Ireland. My father was the oldest child and, like me, he had a gift for basketball. He attended Rice High School, a private parochial school in New York City, on a basketball scholarship. During his freshman year, he made the All-New-York-City Basketball Team, a feat unheard of for a freshman who only stood five-four. Around that same time, my grandfather abandoned my grandmother with six kids, and my father had to quit school to help feed his siblings. He supplemented the family income with money he earned shining shoes on the street corner. My father became very bitter about this and took it out on us every day.

Eight weeks before my eighth-grade graduation, my dad went on one of his binges for four straight days. He called one night and made it verbally clear that he had had enough of my mother and was coming home to do bodily harm to her. You cannot imagine my fright and terror. I knew I had to get her and my sisters out of there quickly. I told my mother that we had to leave because my dad was dangerous at that point and was coming home to kill her. She was speechless but she could see in my face that what he said was true and we could no longer go on living like this night after night.

She reluctantly agreed and with fear in her voice told me to go downstairs and pretend that I was sleeping until he passed out. Fortunately for us, he was so intoxicated when he came home he could hardly walk. We all made believe we were asleep as he staggered in and passed out. Then we loaded up the car with seven garbage bags full of our clothes and left. We began driving to Cape Cod to my Aunt Flo's house. It took us nine long hours because the car kept overheating and we had to stop every half hour to add water to the radiator. My dad never took care of anything except himself, and the car was falling apart from lack of maintenance.

We settled in at my aunt's house and I started school in Cape Cod. I can remember feeling very alone there, once again, as the new kid who didn't know anyone. Only two months remained of my eighth-grade year, therefore, I would be missing graduation back home with my friends. No one noticed me at my new school, so I would go to homeroom then slip out the side door of the school, walk the four miles home, and hide in the sand dunes not far from my aunt's house. Most of the houses where Aunt Flo lived were summer homes, so not a lot of people were around during that time of year.

To pass the time during those long days, I would sneak my basketball out of the house, hide it somewhere outside, and take it with me to school each day. There was a house on a dead-end street nearby that a family only occupied on weekends. I would shoot hoops there for hours and make up imaginary situations in which I was the hero of the game. Thank God I only had two months of school left. Despite the fact that I did not attend much, I managed to do my assignments and graduate eighth grade.

That summer was great. My Uncle John was employed at the local movie theater as a manager. In the summer months, the theater would employ three people to show patrons where to park in the gravel lot. Every day from dusk until the last showing at 9:00 p.m., I took my battery-lit torch and parked cars, or, I should say, showed them where to park. I met some very interesting young people during my employment there. One in particular was Sean, an Irish boy, eighteen years old, traveling across the United States to see the sights. We got along very well. He smoked pot while I parked the cars, but the trade-off was that I got to hear some wonderful tales of Ireland, which I already felt a strong tie to because of my beloved Nanny. Sixty dollars a week was a lot of money for a thirteen-year-old.

My uncle would warn me when R- or even X-rated movies were playing, telling me that I was not to enter the theater. In those days, only one movie would show at a time. When I heard that an X-rated movie was playing, I thought that I might get at least a glimpse of real breasts on the big screen and not in a magazine. I knew exactly what time in the movie that flesh fantasy would happen. Sean and I would sneak in the side door and satisfy our curiosities. The funny thing was that when we would sneak in, my Uncle John would be standing in the back peering through the doors as well. His timing was similar to ours. We kept this going all summer and, in August, Sean and I bid farewell to each other.

My aunt's home was a two-bedroom Cape Cod, maybe a total of twelve hundred square feet, but there were eight people living in it with one bathroom. My mom filed for welfare and housing and was soon approved. We were eventually able to move into a house of our own. We rented a small cape no more than two miles from where my aunt and uncle lived. The house came furnished, so we used what the previous tenants had left for us. On moving day, my mom just sat down on the kitchen chair and began to sob quietly. I knew her heart was shattered; she had no furniture of her own, four children to feed, and was in a home she had never seen before. This was her life now, and I felt the pain she was in even though I was so glad to be away from my father. My room was a heated porch on the side of the house, but I didn't care; it was safe and peaceful. I had my basketball and a hoop, which I had taken with us from New Jersey. I was very happy to be there at first, miles and miles away from my alcoholic father. But after a short while, things in Cape Cod began to deteriorate as well. I knew my mother was in pain. Four kids, no job, on welfare with no belongings to call her own because we had left everything back in New Jersey when we had to flee. I realized how my dad's addictive behavior was ruining her life. All we had was each other, and my mom counted on me daily to help her with my sisters.

Time went on, but I did not make any friends. I just kept shooting hoops all day long. I guess my mom and uncle decided that I needed to make some friends. Without telling me, they signed me up for a youth program at the church to meet kids my own age.

One evening a priest from the church showed up at our house. I was in my room. My mom told me that I had to go with him, and I was very upset about this. I tried to fight, but I did not want to disrespect the priest, and so I reluctantly went with him. We drove to the church hall, and he didn't say a word to me for the entire trip. Once we got to the hall, he led me into a room where there was a gathering of kids, a youth group, of which I knew no one. This made me feel so out of place and embarrassed. Everyone had nice clothes and all I owned were two shirts and two pairs of pants. Being ever so clever at knowing how to hide in uncomfortable situations, I went to the bathroom, climbed out the window and started running toward home. When I tried to walk past this one house in the dark, I got very scared because there was a vicious-sounding dog there. So I stuck out my thumb and started hitchhiking. Wouldn't you know the first car that approached me was the priest? He yelled for me to get in and screamed at me all the way home. From that point on, my uncle and mom never pushed me to do anything like that again.

That summer went by very quickly, and soon school was approaching yet again. I was starting my freshman year of high school. It was a time when most kids are ecstatic about setting out to a new school, a new adventure, and an exciting and care-free chapter in life. That was not the case for me. When I started high school that year, it was like the end of eighth grade all over again. I did not know anyone and the kids were not very friend-ly. Skipping school soon became a normal occurrence for me, only this time school was ten miles from home. Again, I hardly had any clothes and my sneakers had holes in them. I would not skip school every day, but I really could not face it. It would take me three or four hours of walking to get home, but I was in great shape. During gym class, which I always went to, I could outrun and outdistance anyone by so much that the track coach was constantly trying to recruit me. I just never had the confidence or felt the desire to become part of a team. I was afraid someone would find out how I lived or ask about my dad. That fear kept me from trying to get close to the other kids.

When I was alone, I always felt that I was talking to God. I never heard God answer me during those years, but I felt that by talking to Him I was releasing all of the turmoil inside me to someone else. Conversing with God carried me through each day. It made me feel very consoled and relaxed. I was able to think about my problems and work on them. I would sleep during the day on an old go-cart track near my house until school was out. The rich smell of the beautiful pine trees and the sweet sounds of the birds comforted me as I would lay on my back and look up to the sky and daydream about my future and what I would like to do with my life. I was always worried that someone was going to call my mom, yet it was too unbearable for me to attend school every day. The thought of hurting her killed me because my father had done plenty of that and I did not want to add to her burdens. Luckily, my mom never found out.

We did not have many clothes because we had left most of them behind in Vernon Valley. As I said, I only had two shirts for school and two pairs of corduroy pants. The house we rented did not have a washer or dryer, so we washed our clothes in the sink and there were not always clean clothes to wear. Within two weeks of school, I had run out of clean underwear. One day, without thinking about it, I went to take a shower after gym class and left my underwear on the floor by my locker. Bad move. Obviously they were dirty because I was not able to get them washed, and the other kids noticed this and waited around to see who owned them. One guy picked them up and threw them around the locker room, making fun of me. I had never been so humiliated in my entire life. "You wear these?" one of the kids asked. "You're a pig." I put the underwear back on and never went back to that school again. I could not believe I had been stupid enough to let them see my underwear. That is how

I learned to keep things out of sight; then there can be no judgment.

At this point, it was probably about four weeks into the school year. My mom was not feeling well and had to go to the hospital. The diagnosis was a bad gallbladder; she needed surgery. My aunt and uncle took my mom to the hospital and I, as always, stayed with my sisters. I then found out my father had been called and was coming to get us. I felt betrayed by the very people who had saved me so many times before. I had thought we had left him behind for good, but he came the next night and stayed with us. The next day, we packed some things and went to Vernon Valley. We had to stay out of school for a few days, which was a blessing to me. My dad had to go to work and my mom would be in the hospital for three weeks. Each night was like déjà vu. My dad wouldn't come home until 9:00, 10:00, sometimes midnight. Moreover, he would be drunk. My oldest sister had become his housewife, cleaning and cooking, and we both watched our two younger sisters. We soon realized that we were not going back to Cape Cod. My parents had worked things out and, after three weeks or so, my mom was well and she came home to Vernon. We were now all back in our dysfunctional family dwelling.

I realize now that it had been too stressful for my aunt and uncle to take us all back in again, and my mom could not do it all on her own. I love her for the fact that she tried. Overall, our little trip—and our freedom from my father—only lasted five months. When we returned to New Jersey, I moved from my upstairs bedroom to a finished room in the basement. My sisters were getting older and needed their own rooms, and the basement room became my sanctuary. Just closing the door and being on another level of the house helped me cope with the insanity above me.

I transferred to Franklin High School in Sussex County, New Jersey, and seeing all of my old friends again felt good. They had all grown their hair long, and it was funny to see them that way. It really seemed worthwhile to be home again, even if it was with an abusive, alcoholic father. My mom, my sisters, and I had learned how to stay out of my dad's way. My oldest sister continued to be his housewife and we both watched our two younger sisters together.

Christmas was fast approaching, and my mom made it quite clear we had no money for presents. I realized we were all going to pay for our mini-vacation from dad. All I had asked for that year was a basketball. I loved the sport and the escape it represented to me. It was like Tom Hanks and the volleyball that becomes his best friend in the movie *Cast Away*. I woke up Christmas morning and looked under the tree; nothing was there for me, the only gifts were for my sisters. Though I knew my mom did not have money, I was disappointed. When she woke up, she looked at me and said, "That's the best I could do, Billy." When I expressed my surprise at not getting anything, she looked puzzled and replied, "Your father told me he got you a ball." With that, she went into the bedroom and began yelling at him; he had just gotten home four hours earlier and was not exactly full of Christmas cheer. "It's out in the fucking car! Tell him to go get it himself." Upon hearing him yell this, I put on my sneakers, ran outside, and got the basketball. *Merry Christmas to me,* I thought.

We all paid a dear price from that time on. Soon after Christmas, my mom began showing signs that she was pregnant with my fourth sister. Little did I know that her pregnancy had been the reason we had come back from Cape Cod. My mom must have been pregnant when we ran away from my father. She hid her pregnancy very well. My father did not want anymore kids and, since they were strict Catholics, an abortion was out of the question. But my mom knew she could not live on her own with four kids and another on the way. I didn't put it together until recently. I had always thought that my aunt and uncle had let us down; but this truly had not been the case.

In 1971, during my freshman year at Franklin High, I made the school basketball team. Soon, I was considered one of the best players, if not the best, on the team. Being back with familiar faces in school had certainly helped me, and no one knew what had happened to me during those first days at my school in Cape Cod. However, my grades were less than stellar that year. During one practice, my history teacher, who also was the junior varsity basketball coach, came to pay me a visit. In front of all my teammates, he told me that I was failing his class and that school was more important than sports. I stood there looking at him while every eye in the gymnasium was on me. Mortified, to say the least, I wanted to run, but my legs could not move. I felt frozen in place. For a moment, it was as though I was wearing those dirty underpants all over again. I tried to put it out of my mind and, after a few weeks of teasing, I managed to get over it.

Meanwhile, my father's drinking became worse, and he became more and more violent. One day when my mom was eight months pregnant, she asked my dad to bring home a hamburger from the bar for her dinner. He promised to be home by 7:00 p.m. and finally showed up around 11:00 p.m. When he walked in, she was lying on the sofa and she started screaming that it was too late for dinner and she had already eaten. She then told him to take the hamburger and stick it. From my bedroom downstairs, I could hear the heaviness of his footsteps walking toward her. I ran up the stairs, knowing that he was going to hurt her. She started screaming for help and, as I came around the first set of stairs, I could see his left hand around her throat and his other hand shoving the hamburger, still in its bag, into her mouth. As I made it to the top of the stairs, my sisters ran into the living room. They were screaming and crying for him to stop, and I realized at that point that it was up to me to try and stop him.

This drunken maniac, choking his wife, our mother, who was pregnant with his fifth child, suddenly realized our presence and let her go. His focus quickly turned to me as he stood up and asked why I had not tried to stop him. Then he told me, "I know why, because you're not a man. You're a baby, no balls." I looked at him in shock and rage. I wanted to stomp every bit of life out of his body, but I could not move. "How do you hit your own father?" I asked myself. That is when I realized that he wanted me to fight him, and I remembered hearing a story about a confrontation at my Christening between my father and his father. As the story goes, my Uncle John (my dad's brother) made a crack to my grandfather, who then grabbed him by the neck and started punching him. My father saw this going on and said, "You're not hitting any of us anymore." My father then took my grandfather outside and they had a donnybrook. Clearly this violence had been common in my father's family. For the rest of my life, I never feared a man I had problems with, big or small. I knew that, if I had to, if my family was threatened, I could take on anyone. I just could not do anything to harm my father, even when he was hurting us. When I saw that he was going to leave mom alone that night, I retreated to my room as he mumbled some degrading remarks about me under his breath. He was always looking for a reason to engage me in a confrontation, but I would never respond. That went on for the rest of my years at home. These confrontations would continue between the two of us on a regular basis.

As my freshman year ended, I was really excelling in basketball. That summer I played basketball all day long and lost my virginity to alcohol. My first time being drunk was something I will never forget. My best friends at that time were Louie and Herbie, two guys I was with every day. We filled up three glasses of every type of hard liquor Lou's parents had, threw in some ice and chugged. We were hammered in twenty minutes. Lou's parents were at work and we stayed at his house, played music, laughed, and then threw up. Unfortunately for us, Lou's dad had marked the levels of liquor in each of his bottles. Lou got his ass kicked that night, but no one called my parents, so my first attempt at getting high on alcohol was successful.

The summer between my freshman and sophomore years of school, I also learned about the forbidden fruit of intercourse. I was raised Catholic, and my parents did not talk or explain anything to us about sex. Anything I knew I learned from my friends. We all carried condoms in our wallets as people now carry credit cards. Although we had many chances to use them, we did not have the confidence to pull the trigger.

By the time basketball tryouts came around my sophomore year, I had improved dramatically. Not only did I make the basketball team; by the middle of the season, I was starting on varsity. My old freshman coach told me that he had never seen a more improved player in his career. I felt like a million bucks. People were noticing me in school, in the halls and in my classes, not for wearing shitty underwear but for being good at sports. I was getting invitations to senior parties, and it felt weird that people knew my name when I did not know theirs. This would be the case later in my life as well.

Though some things had changed, others had not. Much to my embarrassment, my father would sometimes show up at practice drunk and begin screaming at me in front of my whole team. My teammates would ask me who he was, and I would have to admit that he was my dad.

Nevertheless, my popularity continued into my junior year of high school. The coaches asked me to play football, soccer and track. I also became very close to a boy named John. In 1974, John's family lived in an estate near the high school. His house was beautiful, each room filled with furniture and artwork from all over the world. His parents were divorced and he lived with his father, an airline pilot who had remarried a flight attendant. John's stepmother was a beautiful woman and, when we hung out at his house, I often wished that I was her son.

During that time, my mom started working at night as a telephone operator again. Now that my sisters were older, I no longer had to care for them. I was thrilled about this. After soccer games, I would invite my friends over to drink in my basement. We would watch for the headlights of my mom's car coming up the road, and, when we saw them, everyone would file out the back door and disappear. When my mom got home and saw so many cars leaving, she would ask me who had had a party next door. "Boy, those kids are crazy!" she would say, referring to the boys who lived next door. Meanwhile, she had no idea what had been going on in our house. I managed to pull it off very well, and it felt good that other kids thought I was cool. Unfortunately, alcohol would become a bit of a problem for me by my senior year of school.

When we weren't at my house, John would have a group of us over every weekend since his parents were often away for work. There was a wolf-skin rug in front of a blazing fireplace and a beautiful stereo system in their family room. We had beer, Pink Floyd, and girls—it was truly nirvana for a sixteen-year-old boy. Many kids from school would come over to his parties: the stoners, the brains, and the heavy metal boys. I got to know everyone in school and knew everyone liked me. I enjoyed being with all different kinds of people and, coming from where I did, I never judged anyone.

I inherited the ability to play sports from my father. He was an exceptional athlete. By the end of my junior year, I was not only captain of my basketball team, but also captain of my soccer team. People just seemed to vote for me. This was something that would continue during my years on Wall Street. When we played at other schools, people knew my name from being in the local newspaper. This felt very good, but strange for me. I felt important and accepted at last. In soccer, I played the position of goalie, which was a new spot for me. I made the All Area Team and was the Most Valuable Player on my team. I had been put in charge in many of the things I did, but I could not understand why. I apparently had leadership qualities obvious to everyone but me. I was always chosen in basketball practice to show underclassmen how to shoot a ball properly. College scouts came to see me. I played soccer mostly to stay in shape for basketball, which was my first love.

Basketball season my senior year began with many high hopes for me; however, they would not come to fruition. I was drinking on the weekends, and this news got back to my coach. We were not seeing eye to eye at the time, and all the stress of home life was weighing down on me. I needed to punch back at life since I could not do so to my father. After a game, my team-mates and I went to a friend's house and started popping beers. We had a huge game the next day and, because of the drinking rumors, the coach had followed us. Shortly after, we heard a knock at the door. At that point, I was gunning a beer down my throat while "Highway Star" from Deep Purple was blaring on the stereo. My buddy opened the door and my coach saw every-thing. He threw me off the team the next day. I thought my life was over—no scholarship, no more basketball, no more glory.

Cooler heads eventually prevailed, and I apologized and was put back on the team. We won the State Championship that year and were ranked as the number two team in the state of New Jersey in 1975. To this day, our team holds the record as the school's best. Much to my disappointment, however, I de-veloped a reputation as having disciplinary problems, and col-leges were not recruiting me. But the last shot I took in the

State Championship game was from half court, and I made it. I always thought that was a sign of bigger things to come.

Although I was not able to get an athletic scholarship to college, later in life I played in leagues that had NBA players training in off-season games at the Downtown Athletic Club and was able to hold my own against them. So my dream of playing pro came true in a small way by being able to play against some of these players. That helped me to accept the fact that I had gotten in so much trouble in high school and had made bad choices that had prevented me from going on to college.

# Chapter Three

## *My Wall Street Career*

At the age of eighteen, I had decided that I wanted to work in New York City. Something about the city thrilled me. I am not sure exactly what it was that excited me, but I knew there was money to be made in New York, and I wanted a piece of it. I had many jobs during and after high school, but they were all just a means to get money for gas or to go out and have fun. My whole life, I had always thought about what could make me different from everyone else. I would scan people and situations to see what I could be good at, what my niche in this world would be. I had a feeling I could be successful if I could just get the chance. My personality was engaging, and I always made light of dark situations so other people would feel better. People considered me a leader. I was always voted into those roles although I never asked for or wanted the responsibility. I was captain of my high school basketball and soccer teams, and I had grown used to everyone liking me. I knew from growing up in my alcoholic home how it felt to be embarrassed and to want to crawl in a hole all the time. I never wanted other people to have that feeling.

On St. Patrick's Day after graduation, my sister, her friend and I went into New York City to see the St. Patrick's Day parade. At the time, my father, a former bank teller, was working for a brokerage firm at 120 Broadway. I asked if I could stop in to see where he worked, and he said yes, though he only did so to appease my mother. While in the elevator on the way to my dad's floor, my heart started racing. Something about the atmosphere excited me, although I was not quite sure yet what it was. When I got off the elevator, I immediately saw brokerage rooms full of action. There was yelling and screaming, men watching the numbers on the board like their lives depended on it. The sheer energy in the room gave me goose bumps, and I told myself that I would work in a place like that someday. I didn't know how or why, but I was determined to do it. When I met my father, he barely showed me around and didn't introduce me to anyone before I left. I went home and told my mom about my experience that day, and she later talked to my dad about getting me a job. He told her there was no way, and that I didn't have the brains. To this day, I do not know if he was jealous of me or if he felt threatened that I would do better than he had done. Or maybe he was concerned that, if I worked with him, his coworkers would find out what he was really like. Nothing came out of my visit at the time, but I kept begging my mom to convince my dad to get me a job.

During that year, I worked at a ski resort, a deli, and a gas station, all while living at home. I worked fourteen-hour days between all three jobs. At the ski resort, I worked with a girl named Michele, and we would go out from time to time. One night after work, I drove her home, and she asked me to meet her mom and dad. I agreed and, as we walked into her house, I noticed her sixteen-year-old sister, Kathy, lying on the couch. She immediately caught my attention. Michele brought me upstairs and introduced me to her mom. With that, the phone rang and Michele went to answer it, leaving me to talk with her mother.

At first, our conversation focused on Michele. I explained that I thought Michele was very nice, but that we were not serious. We had been out only a few times and were just friends. Then I turned the conversation to Kathy. Michele's mother told me that her other daughter was dating a guy who was a real loser, and that she wished Kathy would stop seeing him. I don't know what gave me the courage, but I told her mother that I thought Kathy was gorgeous and that I really wanted to take her out. Her mom hinted that this would be okay, and, two days later, I called to ask Kathy out. I asked her if she wanted to take a ride with me to get my stereo fixed. She agreed, and we had a nice talk in the car. At the time, I had lost my glasses and could not afford to get new ones. I thought Kathy was unbelievably beautiful, and, once I had finally replaced my glasses, I could see that she was even more beautiful than I had ever imagined. We began dating and, after two months, I told her she was the one. I knew the first time I saw her that she was the one. I remember praying to God that day, asking Him to let the girl go out with me and promising to make her happy for the rest of my life.

At home, my dad was drinking most of the time but my mom kept talking to him about getting me a job in New York. Finally, that July, he said, "I'll get him in." And he did, though it was a bullshit job that he got me just to appease my mother once again. He told me that if I took this job, I'd be working upstairs in two or three months because his buddy worked up there. I just had to work the entry-level job first. The year was 1977; at nineteen years old, I had my first job on Wall Street as a messenger at Swiss Bank Corporation. It was a menial job. Ninety percent of the people I worked with did not speak English. My dad got me the job just so that his friend, a headhunter, would receive a commission. You only needed a fourth-grade education to get this job. However, my starting salary was $120 a week. Wow! Except I then realized that it would cost $65 a month to commute. Between that and all of my other expenses, I barely broke even, but I knew I had no choice, and my dad told me I would only have to be a messenger for a few months before I moved up.

Each day, I would physically walk stock certificates to banks. I would get on the subway and go to Chase Bank. Then I would go back to Swiss Bank, get another certificate, get back on the subway, and go to another bank to deliver. That is what I did all day long. It was summer, about ninety degrees every day, and, after two months had gone by, I realized that nobody was coming from upstairs to look for me. It was a joke. I would have to get ahead by myself because my father was not going to help me.

I kept my nose in the *Daily News* looking for better positions and, in the late '70s, a lot of firms were looking to hire "brokerage trainees" who could learn the brokerage business. The wonderful thing about this situation was the time frame. The financial markets in New York were rapidly expanding to trading twenty-four hours a day instead of just trading with Europe in the early morning hours and then closing down. All of these overseas companies were trying to open offices in New York City, and so the brokerage business was looking for people who wanted to broker money markets.

I decided to go to a recruiting agency, which would send me on interviews for different brokerage positions that were available. The agency required that everyone take a math test, which consisted of basic addition, subtraction, multiplication, and division. The key was that the tests were timed. You had to answer as many questions as possible and you had to be quick. When I received this test I was confident I could do it. After all, when I was nine years old, my father would beat the answers into my head. Our little study time was pretty intense; I had to get the right answer or my legs would be smacked so hard I would piss my pants. After a while, I learned every one of those timetables backwards and forwards. So when I handed in the agency's test after only a few minutes, it was graded and, of course, all correct. Little had I known it at the time, but those beatings I had taken wound up paying off.

When my perfect scores were confirmed, the head executive from the firm called me in the back for an interview. He was impressed with my high scores and told me he had an opportunity at E. F. Hutton in the commodities department. "Do you know what commodities are?" he asked me. When I told him I had no idea, he told me that the position was for a rip-off clerk. I laughed at the title, and he explained that a rip-off clerk was responsible for ripping off the papers that came out of a teletype machine and putting them down a conveyor belt to people who were sitting at the end of the desks. They would then take the tickets up, file them, and verify the trades executed on the floor of the exchange. The goal was to work your way up and finally make it to the floor of the commodity exchange. Commodities are products that are used in everyday life such as corn, wheat, orange juice, etc. These items are bought and sold on the premise of their values in the future. Every contract that was traded paid a commission to the trading broker. The more contracts that were traded the more money the executing broker made.

I got the job in the commodity department of E. F. Hutton & Company immediately and started at $130 a week. I was so proud of myself—I was finally working for a Wall Street firm! Really, I was only tearing tickets out of a machine and putting them on a conveyor belt. But it was a start, and I remember how proud my mom was of me. "Oh my God, E. F. Hutton, that's a big time job!" she yelled. "You get benefits and everything else."

I guess she was right. I worked in Battery Park Plaza, which was at the end of Wall Street, and I had to wear a suit every day. At the time, I had one suit and I just changed my shirt and tie. Initially, I was going to travel to work with my father. I could not believe that I would have to do this, he appalled me so, but I did not have any money saved up and he traveled into the city each day. I sold my car so I could save on the loan payment and auto insurance. I felt like I had no choice.

It did not take long before commuting together to Wall Street became a disaster because my father continued to drink every day. We would usually meet at the train station and drive home together when we got to our stop. The commute was a bitch. We lived in Sussex County, and so it was almost a two-hour commute on a good day—an hour on the train and a 45-minute drive from the station. My father was used to drinking every night, so it pissed him off that he had to cut short his playtime to meet me after work. The plan was to catch the 5:30

train to come home. Fifty percent of the time, he did not show up. I would call my mom and ask where he was. She wouldn't be able to get a hold of him though because he was already at the bar, and so she would tell me to just get on the train and wait for him at the station. I wanted to bust the goddamn glass out of the telephone booth, and she was as distraught about it as I was. She would softly say, "I can't get a hold of him." I knew it killed her that I had to wait there for him so many times. Looking back, I realize that I was the unwilling participant in a silent battle of wills between my parents. My mother believed that my commuting with my father would force him to stop drinking after work and come home. My father thought I would be glad to start hanging with him and his friends in the bar after work and enable him to continue his pattern.

One winter evening, it was freezing out and I had no way to get home from the train station, so I called Kathy to pick me up. She had just gotten her license, and her mom's car was not in the best condition, but she came to get me. If she had not come, I would have had no way home that night, as my father did not get home until after two a.m.

After Kathy dropped me off that night, I realized that I needed my own car. It was time for me to make a break from my father. I searched around and found a blue Ford Pinto. I financed almost the whole amount—$2900—which put me at a loss per month from what I made to what I owed. My monthly train ticket was $65, and now I would be paying $90 per month for my car loan. Between gas and other living expenses, I just about broke even. However, it was so much better being able to control my own movements.

I was still living at home, but I finally took a stand with my father. I had to borrow $100 from him to get the car and I told him I'd pay him back the minute I had the money. On a Saturday two weeks after he had given me the loan, he and my mom were arguing and I walked by them to go upstairs. I told him to leave her alone and knock it off. That took the attention off my mom. "Where's my money?" he asked. When I told him I didn't have it, he replied, "What else is fuckin' new? This is bullshit. I told you I want that goddamn money." He was practically spitting in my face.

"What are you going to do, make me pay the bills around here like you make her do?" I asked. Before I could even finish my sentence, he was coming toward me as though he was going to hit me. This was what he had been waiting for his whole life. I was standing in front of the main door of our bi-level house. As he came down the stairs, my sisters, who were standing at the top of the steps, screamed at my dad not to hit me. I, being naïve, said, "Don't worry, he's not gonna hit me." I was not trying to be cocky; I was trying to calm things down. The next thing I knew, he hit me and I went airborne right through the screen door. I fell back on my head. I was dazed and, as I tried to get up I could see him through the door standing there just waiting for me to retaliate. I was frozen in place. *This is my father. You don't hit your father,* I thought. I pulled myself together, got up, and refrained from hitting him. At that very moment, I became a man.

Though it was difficult to leave my mom and my sisters, I got in my car and left, not once looking back. I drove to Kathy's house. She had six brothers and sisters and lived in a modest middle-income home. I did not know what to do. Her dad was a wonderful man. I explained the situation to him and he said that I was welcome to stay there for as long as I needed. Again, as I look back on my life, I feel there was always someone watching out for me from above.

Kathy was sixteen and I was nineteen. We had been seeing each other for two and a half months. At nineteen years old, I was on my own. I had no clothes, just my car and a sleeping bag, which I used as my bed each night on the cement floor of my girlfriend's basement. My mom called me and, though she felt bad, she did not encourage me to come home. She understood that I could not live in the same house with my dad anymore. After a week, I told my mom I was never coming home again, and I realized she already knew. My father, however, fully expected me to flop and come home and kiss his ass. I guess he had done a better job at making me a man than he thought. My mom and I did not speak much over the next couple of years. It was too uncomfortable because I felt she betrayed me by siding with my dad and not fighting for me to stay.

As the months passed, Kathy graduated from high school and got a job in an office. I knew I really had to push myself at work because I needed to make more money. I continued to get up at five a.m. It was wearisome in the beginning, with no bedroom and no privacy, but Kathy's house felt more like home than my home had because I was not under the constant scrutiny of my father. Her parents really did treat me like a son.

Kathy and I finally saved up enough money to find our own apartment. We were trying to cut our lengthy commutes down; I was still doing my usual two-hour commute and she was driving 50 minutes. We moved to Newfoundland, New Jersey, where she could walk to work and I was only ten minutes from the train station. We had no furniture and borrowed random pieces from family members. Kathy's parents, strict Catholics, understood the situation but wanted us to get married sooner rather than later. Kathy's father stopped by after work one evening and asked us to please go to a priest and get married. I sold my stereo and used the money to buy Kathy a modest engagement ring.

Kathy came from a family of seven children who were all still at home. We knew that her parents could not afford to pay for any kind of wedding reception for us. My mother said that she and my dad would try to make something happen at the local VFW hall. (Of course, I was thinking this should have been free for all the money my dad had spent there over the years). My sister Connie came over and sat down with Kathy and Kathy's mom to develop the guest list. The next day, Kathy's mom called and asked if they could add more guests to the list, and she generously offered to pay for them. At this point, my mother had still not asked my father to throw the party. Both sides of the family started arguing about who should pay for what. After a very miserable attempt by both families to organize a wedding for us, Kathy and I decided to get married at the courthouse. Kathy's parents and my mother came, along with my ten-year-old sister. Once we were married, my mother congratulated us and then said she had to run home for the birthday party she was throwing for my sister. My in-laws took us out to dinner at a local restaurant. Years later, I bought Kathy a $3,000 engagement ring, but she never let me forget that she had not had a traditional wedding and honeymoon, and I felt guilty about that every day of our married life.

Meanwhile, my job in commodities was slowly improving, and now I had some experience in trading markets. However, in order to get into the brokering pit to trade, you needed a college degree in finance. I worried that I would never be able to trade and began to wonder if I was wasting my time. But trading—the screaming and yelling and price changes—I just loved it! It had now been two years since my father threw me out. I had begun to talk to my mom regularly, and my dad was always inquiring as to how I was doing at work. I then got the idea that, if I quit my job on the commodity floor, my dad would feel bad because of all he had done to me in the past and get me an interview in one of the companies where he had contacts. At least that is what I was hoping. By doing this, I could then become a trading broker without a college degree, a position I had not been able to reach at my previous company. This would be a truly outrageous move considering the first job my dad had gotten me, but my gut instinct told me it would be different this time because I was no longer "green."

With that thought in mind, I pulled the trigger and quit my job. Kathy was absolutely beside herself, and she let me know it. We had no savings and could not afford to live on her salary alone. However, I just had this feeling inside. The next day I told my mom that I had quit and, sure enough, my dad called me to ask what had happened. I had not seen my dad in two years. He had not come to my wedding and had made no contact in that time. I gave him a roundabout story as to why I quit, to which he replied, "Wait a minute. Don't snow the snowman.

I don't want any bullshit." I explained to him that I was not happy doing what I was doing and felt commodities were a dead end. Again, the truth paid off, as my dad responded, "Yeah, I heard about that with commodities. Look, there is this company opening up and I know this guy, Lou. Call him Monday and I'll see what I can do."

The next day I called Lou and got an interview to see a British man named Robert. He told me to come in the next day between noon and one o'clock. I eagerly arrived at eleven forty-five and, as I was knocking on the door, Robert came out and remarked sternly, "I told you after noon." Meanwhile, I could hear people screaming inside his office and I wondered what the hell was going on in there. Robert explained that the company was international, which meant they were trading with Europe and the market would calm down at noon. Then he told me to sit down and wait. Once it was past noon, he took me into his office. He asked about my dad and my experience in commodities, then about why I wanted to trade.

"Ever since I was in my dad's office a few years ago and got a taste of this kind of work, I've had a hunger for it," I replied. "There is something invigorating about it. I would love to become a broker." He hired me on the spot, saying he'd start me at $12,000. So there I was, in my early twenties and making $12,000 a year. That was a very successful salary for a trainee back then. When I went home and told Kathy, she was both relieved and elated.

Each day I had to watch these huge boards with figures scrolling across them as the guys yelled out numbers, and I had to write those numbers down. If you did not hear them, you got your ass chewed out. The trick was listening to four or five conversations at a time and determining which information was pertinent. After several months, I could not take it anymore. If I didn't hear the numbers right or put them on paper incorrectly, these men would call me "asshole," "stupid," or "jerk-off." Each person felt that I was exclusive to him. I refused to put up with it. Because of my upbringing, I did not possess the qualities I needed to withstand the daily verbal abuse. Every time someone would yell at me, which was part of the job, I saw my father's face. After six months, I came home yet again and told Kathy that I could not do it anymore. She told me I couldn't quit, but I quit anyway.

## Chapter Four

# *Mastering the Trade*

I was out of a job for two months, and so Kathy and I moved back in with her parents. I loved her father. He welcomed us with open arms. One month into my hiatus, my father-in-law, who was a Port Authority Police Lieutenant, came home while I was sitting in the living room watching a movie. He looked at me and said, "Don't get splinters in your ass, Bill!" It took me a few minutes to figure out what he was saying, but his point soon rang loud and clear. I never wanted to lose his approval. The man had no idea that inside I was struggling to continue my marriage.

Through our early days together, I could not get enough of Kathy. We had similar values and I thought we wanted the same things out of life. The problem was that she only wanted to be with me. I, on the other hand, was very outgoing and had many friends. This caused a great deal of problems between us, and I wasn't ready to isolate myself from the rest of the world. I got tired of it very quickly. I felt smothered and probably didn't realize how dysfunctional I was behaving, having seen my parent's display of marriage. Everything was so stressful for me that I panicked and wanted out from it all. So I choreographed our move back with Kathy's parents so that when I left her, she would not be alone. This was not the healthiest thing, I know. But Kathy was not happy when I went out with my friends, and I felt suffocated.

Kathy's father never made me feel like a burden. One evening, however, he took me for a ride and told me I needed to get my act together, get a job, and take care of my wife. Although I was not happy in my marriage, I knew I had to get back to work.

After that talk, I called a former coworker and asked for help in getting another job. The man said he would see what he could do, but two weeks went by and I didn't hear anything. In the meantime, Kathy was working at Prudential as a secretary, and her parents did not like that she was working while I was not. Then my old coworker finally called back and said he knew a company that needed a link man, the person responsible for exchanging prices back and forth over the phone to overseas offices. I called and set up an interview. As luck would have it, my meeting went well and they offered me the job at a salary of $16,000 a year. In addition, they were going to send me to London for a week to meet my new colleagues. It happened that fast.

Meanwhile, Kathy continued to manipulate and control me. She would not let me play basketball or hang out with my friends. I was to be either at work or at home, and if I dared to want to do anything different from this routine, she would tell me that I never put her needs first. I just could not figure out what to do or where to go. I was very frustrated both personally and in my career. But I thought this new job opportunity would allow me the chance to get things back on track with her and find fulfillment through my work.

Soon I was on my way to JFK to board a flight to England. My mother-in-law and father-in-law joked with me about my stellar interviewing skills, but Kathy was not happy about my leaving. On our way to the airport, she became sick to her stomach. We thought it was a flu bug.

The flight to London was my first time on an airplane. The flight lasted six hours, and I tried to stay calm as I headed into a new country where I didn't know anyone. I stayed at the Tower Hotel on the River Thames and was scared and lonely. I had a new job and would be meeting my new employers in the morning. I had carte blanche to spend money on whatever I needed. That week was very eye-opening for me. I was treated to great restaurants courtesy of my colleagues and was, in general, treated like a king. I was also able to see how the market started in Tokyo and worked its way to London and then eventually to New York. It all came so fast, and I was trying to absorb what was happening to me. It was an adventurous and extremely informative week to say the least. I made some very good friends and learned about big business.

When I arrived home one week later, a much worldlier person, I had learned that there were different cultures that I had never known existed. I went back to work and started my job with a new sense of confidence. Kathy's stomach ailment continued to bother her, and we realized it was probably not the flu. She went to see her doctor and found out she was pregnant with our first child. When I came home that evening, she told me the news. The day I found out that I was going to be a father was the most influential day of my life. I knew there were issues with our relationship; however, I swore my child would never want for anything and that I would be the best father ever. We immediately decided that Kathy would stay home and raise our baby.

My next move was to make up for the loss of her salary. It was then that I began to understand that the higher your pay, the more intense your job. What looked wonderful on bank checks every two weeks was hell on me at work. The verbal abuse left me so frustrated and angry I really wanted to kill people. It was a pressure cooker in that office from seven a.m. until five p.m. Traders screaming, people so stressed to make brokerage; it was hell. This went on for months and, although I was making more money, I was a nervous wreck.

That Christmas season, Kathy and I were living in a nice apartment and we had just finished decorating our Christmas tree. At eight months pregnant, she had felt some cramping and mild pains earlier in the day and, that night, we went to the hospital. She was in labor for sixteen hours and, on the morning of December 7, 1980, our daughter Marie was born. I was in the birthing room with Kathy, and watching my daughter come into the world gave me the most unbelievable feeling. I held that child when she was just seconds old and I could not believe that she had just been inside my wife. That moment is forever etched in my mind.

Back at work, I was approaching my six-month probation period. I had a company credit card, which all brokers received to entertain representatives of large accounts. I asked for permission to use it personally and purchased tickets for Kathy and me to go to the Virgin Islands. I had always felt bad that I had not been able to give her a honeymoon when we got married. My company gave me the okay and off we went for one week to St.

Thomas. Marie was six months old now and stayed with Kathy's parents. When we flew over those islands, I didn't think it was possible to see such clear, turquoise water. On the island, I took a deep breath and inhaled the lush, green, tropical paradise. I felt wonderful to be able to give Kathy that week; after all, she had given me a beautiful daughter.

At this time, the corporate heads in my company were brokers from across the pond because the company's headquarters were in England. They were coming over to the states and, by 1980, everything was starting to go "global." We were now trading twenty-four hours a day. The European companies would send their top men over to open branches in New York. Each of these individuals had his own idea of how he wanted to groom his protégés. Most of the men hired now were college educated. I worked with one man from Notre Dame and others who had graduated from Penn State; everyone had either a math degree or a degree in economics. This caused frustration for me because, with only a high school diploma, I did not have the advanced math aptitude my new coworkers did.

Though well-educated, however, some of these men had had an upbringing in London similar to mine in New York City. They would yell vulgar, belligerent street talk at me. I was under extreme pressure because if I made one mistake I could lose thousands of dollars for the company. Back when I was on the "link line" shouting out prices, my colleagues were under the gun to make money and they would throw their markers at me yelling, "You're a piece of shit. Get my prices down that line now!" I was being treated like garbage again. Day in and day out, I was the voice of 50 plus people to my offices overseas.

Trying to transform their anxiety-ridden behaviors into cash was overwhelming. At home, my internal alarm clock always went off around five a.m., and I would find my daughter peacefully sleeping in her crib before I would shower for work. I would feel a total knot inside, knowing that I had another day of abuse ahead. Because of this, I kept changing jobs. However, you cannot quit when you have a wife and a child and there is nowhere else to go. But I was not going to take the belittlement either.

Once again, it felt as though someone was looking down on me. A gentleman named Steve, a colleague who had left our company to open a similar firm for another group of investors, unexpectedly called and offered me a job. And it was not only a job, but a job with a salary of $40,000 a year. I must have impressed Steve with my personality and my ability at some point. After hanging up the phone, I wanted to jump through the roof.

Three years later, Kathy became pregnant again, and my beautiful son, Scott, was born. The year was 1983, and I truly loved my wife and kids. My insecurities from the early stage of our marriage were gone. I loved providing for my family—a very important picture in my personal photo album. In 1985, I transitioned from a link man to a broker with Tradition North America. I had a very tough position. Now speaking directly to the banks, I had to entertain my accounts and show them my appreciation for their business. This meant going to the best restaurants for dinner or lunch and cocktails, always cocktails. With alcoholism in my genes, I became at risk. Although I was drinking more, I learned how to structure my alcohol consumption. Cocaine was the drug of choice when going out with accounts back then. It was an appetizer on a menu, mostly a starter course that kept people awake after a long day. I knew if I got attached to that remedy it would ruin my career.

When you make a lot of brokerage, a sizable expense account allows you to eat in any of the top restaurants in the city. I had special places I would take my clients, where the staff knew me and what I wanted to order. When there were lines to get in, we were brought to the front, seated, and waited on immediately. I knew this was not reality and just enjoyed being in the limelight as long as it lasted. I was a twenty-nine-year-old high school graduate making $75,000 a year. I had bullshit my way to the top and still had no idea what I was doing. People liked me, and I learned the brokerage game well enough to play. "You know, he's a nice guy. He's got two kids at home, we'll give him a little bit here and there," my accounts would say. Even scrounging, I was able to make a good salary. Yet I never lost my awareness of what it was like to have nothing, and my past was always on my mind.

Soon, Kathy and I wanted a house, so we began looking near Little Silver, New Jersey. I knew that I needed to be near a train station in order to get to work, and the area seemed perfect. We found a beautiful Cape Cod-style home that cost $130,000. I almost had a cardiac arrest at the price, considering my parents had paid only $18,000 for their home, but Kathy assured me that my salary was more than adequate for the mortgage payment. She took care of all our finances and I trusted her. All I wanted was to make her happy.

Shortly after that, I began drinking every day to help me deal with the stress I was experiencing. I was slowly killing myself inside trying to give Kathy and the kids the best life possible. I began to make excuses for going for a drink after work. Most times it was just to talk with the guys about all the stress of the house and job and not making enough brokerage for work, where the pressure was unbelievable. I was fighting my way tooth and nail to get to the top. I still had not mastered my trade. College graduates were all around me. I just followed everyone else until I secured an account. I had bought a home in a great neighborhood and had everything going for me: a wife and two beautiful children. Despite my hatred for my father and my determination not to become him, I could not help it. I was sliding downhill rapidly and really had to search my soul. "Wait a minute, I'm becoming an alcoholic," I remember saying aloud. Those very words coming out of my mouth made me look into the mirror and see my greatest fear. I was becoming my father. "No way," I said, "This is going to stop today." Unfortunately, my words weren't strong enough to keep my actions in check.

At work, my problems did not go unnoticed. I was just picking up the phones and going through the motions. Finally, it all came crashing down. The company I was working for was not making money, so they sent one of their top men over from England to come in and clean house. He came in, looked over contracts and deals, and sat down next to everyone's desk to see how they were performing. One day he came over to my area, looked at me, and noticed that I was not meeting my quotas. He called me in the back and immediately cut my salary by $15,000. I went home and told Kathy I was going to quit. She told me I couldn't. I knew she was right. I would have to find another job before I pulled the trigger for the umpteenth time.

A good friend of mine got me an interview at Euro Brokers and that is where I met my mentor, Charlie Johnston.

Euro Brokers hired me at $60,000 a year, again because of my personality and my ability to communicate with others. But it was not long before I started waffling there. I continued to drink heavily because I knew I was not meeting my ratios, which were supposed to be three times my annual salary in production. For example, if you made $100,000, you had to bring in $300,000 in commission from assorted accounts. My department head decided he would contact my accounts to get their approval on releasing me from my duties to them. But all my clients told him that if he fired me, they would pull their accounts. I don't know how I had earned their support; I had never known they felt so strongly about me. As a result of the feedback from my accounts, Charlie Johnston, Senior Vice President of the company, came over to me, put his hand on my shoulder, and said, "Bill we're going to take a chance on you, laddie." He told me I would be sitting next to him for the next nine months and that he would teach me the market. He was a wonderful Scottish fellow with a huge heart, and that man sat beside me for the next nine months and taught me those markets inside and out. It all started to click for me by the beginning of 1987, and, with Charlie's help, the fog cleared. From then on, I really understood the market and all that it entailed. Until that point, I had been a third-string player in the business. Now I understood the mechanics and everything fell into place. I knew what would happen in the market and successfully steered my accounts. I became a leader instead of a follower in the markets. I will always be in Charlie's debt.

After a full year of his training, I had also stopped the boozing and started to work out. I was feeling more confident now both physically and mentally. I had found my niche and had the chance to make myself known. I started to pursue all of the big accounts that would not deal with our firm, either because they didn't have a relationship with anyone there or because they thought our markets were not that strong. I began coming in early every morning and cold calling, which is calling a bank and trying to get someone to listen to your proposal. These firms already had brokers, but I would ask for favors from my other accounts, requesting that they give me exclusive pricing for the new clients I was trying to list. It was tough, but I stayed with it, and eventually the banks started to answer my calls. Within a year, I was promoted to Vice President. I was now making over $100,000 a year in addition to a $40,000 bonus, and I was well on my way up the ladder. I was in charge of my area, gave brokering classes to the new recruits, and was now the teacher instead of the student. I had made it thanks to Charlie, who had become a very good friend and mentor. Thankfully, Charlie retired prior to September 11, so he was not a witness, or like so many others, a victim.

At home, Kathy became disenchanted with our Cape Cod home in Little Silver. She felt it was too small for us. We had just purchased a new Volvo sedan and now "needed" a larger home to park it in front of. I loved that house very much and would have been content to live there forever. I still go back sometimes to see the home and neighborhood and reminisce about my life and family and how it was back then. We moved to Middletown, New Jersey, only four miles away. It was a bigger house with lots of room, and now there was remodeling, too. Overall, we put $90,000 into the house (on top of a $325,000 mortgage), from the driveway and landscaping to new mantels, molding and carpeting. The only thing we left alone was the kitchen.

At the age of 33, I had a reputation at work for "moving the markets," and I had become one of the top producers in my firm. Offers from other companies began to come in, but I was very content where I was and comfortable in my surroundings. I could not believe I had such a wonderful situation with work and my family. We were now settled in an upscale neighborhood living in a beautiful home. I was so proud every time I walked in the door of my house. But there was a lot going on inside that house that I wasn't aware of.

From the beginning of our marriage, I had given my wife full control of the finances. I did not want to deprive her of money like my father had done to my mother. That decision would destroy me financially in the end. Although I eventually made an annual salary in excess of $300,000, I had no idea Kathy had never saved a dime. She spent our money relentlessly, all the while reassuring me that she was saving. Years later, I would find very expensive items, like dozens of Lenox pieces and other collectibles, still in their packages, seemingly purchased for no reason at all. She would buy furniture and decide later on that she did not like it, and I would come home to find that she had given it all away.

One evening I arrived home to find the landscaper who had previously done some work for us, planting six new twelve-foot high pine trees on the property line between our house and our neighbor's. They were putting in a swimming pool next door and Kathy felt they were over the property line that separated our parcels. Without any thought to what she was doing, Kathy took it upon herself to stick a metal rod in the ground like a surveyor and claim her property. Obviously, it was not the right place. When my neighbors saw this, they were furious. They called Kathy over and verbally lambasted her. That prompted Kathy to put the trees in that very afternoon. When I opened my car door and asked what was happening, the grounds worker was probably wondering why I didn't know about the project. He looked at me and just continued to dig. The final cost for the job was $6,000. This behavior toward all of our neighbors continued over the years. Slowly, we became estranged from most of the people in our development. Kathy had accomplished nothing positive. The tree barrier that was now between our neighbors and us physically represented the chasm that would continue for many more years to come.

In the meantime, another firm was aggressively pursuing me. They wanted me to leave Euro Brokers and join their company. Word got out about my potential departure, and Charlie, in an attempt to head off any further talks, flew in a very old colleague of mine, Ian, who was now working for Euro Brokers in England. I trusted this man very much. That is a rarity in the business. One Sunday morning, I heard a knock at my front door. When I opened it, I saw my friend Ian smiling at me. "Hey, mate!" he said. I just stared at him in disbelief. When I asked what he was doing there, he said, "I hear you may be leaving us and we're here to stop that." "We?" I asked. He looked at me and said, "Yes, Charlie and I. He's sitting in the car in your driveway. May we come in?" At this point Kathy had come to the door and the kids were running around looking for breakfast. I looked outside and there was Charlie, sitting in his Jaguar waving at me. They both came in and, after a lengthy chat, offered me an in-ground swimming pool, the lease of a BMW convertible, and a $60,000 pay raise on the condition that I continued to work for Euro Brokers.

I had to pinch myself after they left. Kathy and I were both in disbelief that this was happening to a poor kid from the Bronx. I never told anyone at work about the deal to keep me on, but rumors flew. Unfortunately, as I continued to work there, other colleagues became extremely jealous and caused much grief for me by not covering as coworkers do whenever I went on a vacation or was out of the office. It became a very difficult work atmosphere. The next July, I came back after a week's vacation to find that my peers had not serviced any of my accounts. My clients were furious and could not believe that no one was backing me up when I was not in the office. After that incident, I realized how quickly people turned on me when they believed they were not getting all the benefits that I was.

# Chapter Five

## *February 1993*

In February 1993, Euro Brokers was still my place of employment. My office was on the 31st floor of the North Tower of the World Trade Center. On February 26th, dark gray clouds filled the sky, and it was cold and snowy. I had just made my daily lunchtime call to Kathy. We tried to chat every day around noon so that we could confer as to what was going on at work and at home. All of a sudden, I heard a loud boom and could feel a strong vibration under my feet. The whole building shook. My wife said that the TV had just blinked. My colleagues and I sat there wondering what had just transpired. We did not know it at the time, but a bomb had just exploded on the first level of the parking garage. Terrorists were not on anyone's mind at that point, and terrorism was not something that happened on United States soil. There were no announcements of any kind, and people were calling in to tell us a bomb had gone off downstairs after seeing live television coverage from outside the tower. We were told nothing by building management; there were no alarms, nothing. A few of my friends ran to the window only to see a light mist and snow flurries. I continued to speak to my wife as my friend, Mike, looked out the window and said, "I'm getting out of here. Maybe a plane hit the building." He did not know that he was eight years early on that call. My wife said I had better leave, but I told her I couldn't—I had work to do. Finally, she convinced me to go; however, I took my sweet time.

People in the office began to slowly leave their desks. I said goodbye to my wife and hung up the telephone. I picked up my wallet and got my coat, in no big hurry. I walked into the hallway with Mike, and we immediately realized something was terribly wrong. A very thin layer of bluish smoke hovered around the ceiling. My first thought was to take the elevator, but Mike said we should take the stairs in case there was a fire. We had no idea what was about to unfold.

When we entered the stairwell, everything appeared to be calm. People were descending slowly at first. As we began to make our way down, the smoke got very thick, making it difficult to see and breathe. Mike, a stockier man, was sweating profusely and gasping for air. I, on the left side, could feel the banister and kept my hand on it. We descended with three men across each stair as we walked down. Mike was in the middle and a British colleague, Colin, was on the right. Remembering school fire drills from when I was young, the railing in my left hand served as a non-visual guide while we continued down the stairs. This way if anyone pushed or shoved me, I could maintain my balance. The banister also told me where the stairs stopped and started as we came to each floor.

The lighting was sparse in the stairwell and all we could do was follow the voices of the people below us. It began to get more and more crowded and people were starting to push forward. At each floor, more people were trying to get out, and our progress slowed to a crawl. As we continued to proceed downward, we could hear screaming from the levels below. We were walking over shoes that people had kicked off and purses that had been discarded. Mike held my arm and together, we maintained our position of three across the stairs. The smoke and heat were getting worse on each succeeding floor. We thought about getting off, but the doors to each level were automatically locked from the inside. This was done as a security measure so no one could enter onto the floors at night. We had no choice but to continue to walk down.

The further down we got, the more people were steadily streaming into the stairwell and piling into the massive chain of humanity pushing their way down. Although the elevators were forbidden in emergencies such as this, I was tempted to push through a nearby door and see if that would be a more viable option.

By now, there were hundreds of people in the stairwells. It was getting hotter. People were starting to lose control. Some were screaming and trying to push ahead out of sheer panic and fear. When we lost what minimal lights we had, it caused a frenzy of pushing and shoving. At that point, each of us could only guess what was going on. "Keep holding on!" I yelled to Mike as I took my tie off and wrapped it around my mouth and nose so I could breathe through the smoke. I did not want to go down. "We're going into a fire!" I yelled. I was petrified that we were walking into an incinerator below. Whether that was the case or not, I risked being trampled from behind if I froze.

As we continued to walk, the screams got louder and louder and the smoke was overwhelming. The taste of burning metal and sulfur overpowered my senses. My chest felt so heavy I could not bear to breathe as I pressed my tie tightly against my mouth in an attempt to block the smoke. People were screaming and yelling, "Please, go faster!" Others continued to discard their belongings on the steps. Some people were falling down and some just could not catch their breath.

It seemed like we were in the stairwell for hours, but finally we could hear firefighters yelling for us to go to the lights they were waving at the bottom of the stairs. When we reached the bottom, there was chaos all around us. A firefighter at the end of the stairwell was screaming, "Walk to the light!" He continued to wave his light around in an effort to guide us through the thick smoke.

After going through the door near the firefighters, I had no idea where I was. Breathing was a struggle now due to the thick, dark smoke. All I could see was a very small strip of daylight on the ceiling, which I knew was coming from outside. That is what I focused on. I was determined to get to that spot as quickly as possible. Eventually, that light led us all out. When I finally walked outside, I could not believe my eyes. To my left was the parking garage, and a large plume of black smoke was billowing out of the entrance. Fire trucks and ambulances were everywhere. Firefighters were on their knees crawling into the garage, feeling the ground to determine where the cement dropped off beneath them. That picture will be in my mind forever. *This is a movie,* I said to myself. *It's not real. It cannot be.*

I looked at Mike and all the other people who were walking out of the tower, everyone covered in black soot, two lines of black carbon coming down from each nostril. We had breathed it in so heavily that it coated the insides of our noses and was choking our throats. We were all in shock. Terror and chaos were all around us now. I could see my friend Vince walking out behind me, terror on his face as well. He was holding his hand over his mouth and nose and he was crying. None of us knew at that time how close we had just come to being murdered. The terrorists had fully expected that tower to topple into the other, and we the victims had had no idea what was unfolding.

The three of us crossed the street and stood there trying to figure out what had just transpired. Everyone had stopped right outside the entrance to World Trade Center One. Some people were bleeding and others were passing out from the stress and heavy amounts of smoke and soot. I looked up at the building and heard glass breaking above me. Others started screaming that the building was falling down, so I started running with the crowd. Mike, Colin and I turned right and proceeded to run toward the waterfront. I felt like I was part of a human herd of cattle on a dead run. If you did not move with the herd, you would be trampled. People just reacted. Instinctively, you do not care about anything other than saving yourself.

As I began to run, I headed for the water; I figured if the tower was going to come down, at least I'd be able to jump into the Hudson River. It was a mad scramble for cover. I prayed that if the building was falling, it would not fall in my direction. I was waiting to hear the metal twist and tear apart as the building fell. The feeling was like nothing I had ever experienced before. I soon realized that the noise of breaking glass was coming from people who were still in the building, breaking windows in an effort to breathe. The building was not coming down. We stopped running and just looked at each other thinking about how we could have died. My heart was pounding, and Mike looked like he was very close to having a heart attack.

After a little more walking, we finally made it to the ferry and crossed over to Jersey City. My two friends and I took three shots of Jack Daniels each from the closest bar, still trying to figure out what had just happened across the water. None of us spoke much; we were dazed and still couldn't believe that what had happened was caused by a bomb. Inside the bar, the television was on and we regrouped as much as possible. I listened to the radio on the way home and heard there were people trapped in the upper floors calling 911 for help. I just could not comprehend that someone had tried to kill any of us. In later months, we learned that the terrorists had come very close to achieving their goal. If the bomb had blown upwards instead of down, the one building would have fallen into the other, just as they had planned.

After the bombing, we were all called back to work the following Monday. Our office had been temporarily relocated to 7 World Trade Center in the Solomon Business office while they cleaned up the damage in our building. A few weeks later, we were allowed to go back to our old office to clean out our desks and personal belongings. When I walked onto the 31st floor, I began to shake inside. As I entered my office, it was like that day had been frozen in time; it was 12:15 all over again, as if I was in a time capsule. Old cups of coffee and half-eaten sandwiches were on the desks, pictures of children and wives were still on display, and the board we used to put prices on each day was exactly as we had left it. It was a very surreal experience. "They" had tried to kill us, but why? Why would anyone want to kill innocent people? At that point, I really did not have a choice about going back to work. I had a family, a large mortgage, and bills comparable with my lifestyle. I knew my friends didn't have a choice either. But none of us wanted to die at work. That experience left a mark on me. The glory I felt from my success was now overshadowed by a strong feeling of insecurity and doubts about my safety.

It had already been determined prior to the bombing that Euro Brokers would be leasing new space on the 84th floor. It was almost three-quarters of the way complete when the bomb went off. We were moving because our lease had expired and Euro's owners wanted to keep the prestigious address of the World Trade Center. After the bombing, not many companies were fighting for space in the building, so the ones that did stay were receiving quite good offers on new leases. When our offices finally moved, we found we now had to take two sets of elevators to get to our new floor. I knew I was not alone in feeling uneasy about this location farther away from the ground level. The 31st floor had taken us 45 minutes to escape using the stairs. I had a bad feeling about switching elevators. In time though, we all learned to adapt with a heightened sense of awareness. The offices were new, the carpeting was nice and, before long, we were on top of the world again, trading during the day and dining with our clients at night.

The summer of 1993 was unusually hot and humid, and the electrical power grid of lower Manhattan was at peak output. One day, we were all trading as usual when, around 1:00 p.m., a generator that was located down on Wall Street overheated. We heard a huge explosion and the lights went out. The entire ground shook again. I never saw so many people get up and run for the doors in my life. We were now experienced in the field of terrorism and conditioned to make very quick exits. I knew then that the 84th floor was not for me.

My annual July vacation was coming up. I always took off the week of my birthday, July 5th. That year, we decided to rent a house in Cape Cod. We even brought our dog, Scottie, and had a great time. I tried not to think about the bombing, or having to scramble away from my desk again, but I could not put the thought of having to go back into that building out of my mind. I had a very uneasy feeling about it.

When I returned from vacation, the city had placed concrete barriers around all the entrances to the World Trade Center so that no one could drive into the building. It was very intense to see those concrete walls everywhere. They created a feeling of fear instead of security. By midweek, I realized my colleagues had not properly serviced my accounts while I was away, and I received many complaints from my clients. This had been an ongoing issue since my agreement with Charlie to stay. Between this and the fear of another bombing, I just had to get out of that tower. My head felt like it was in a vice with all the people around me screaming prices and brokering for trades. All of a sudden, it seemed like madness. I decided to resign. Although I admired my boss and hated leaving the company that had made me a star, I finally sat down and wrote my resignation letter. I put the letter in an envelope, handed it to a friend, and walked out. In the elevator, I thought, *What am I doing? I have two kids, a high mortgage and car payments, and I just quit.*

My trip home from work that day was a blur; my mind wandered everywhere and I felt sick inside. When I arrived home, my wife was on the phone with Charlie, my boss, and he agreed that it was probably time to part ways. I had one year left on my contract, but we negotiated a deal where I would sit out of the market for three months. It was a normal scenario for people who had valid contracts with time left. I immediately decided that I would take my family back to Cape Cod for another week. The kids knew nothing of my resignation and they loved the fact that we were going back to the ocean. For three months, I received full salary, my car payment, and expense money. I knew that it would not be too difficult to get another job offer.

We asked Kathy's parents to join us for the week, and at first they said no but then decided to come and spend three days with us. My father-in-law was a joy to have around and the kids loved their grandpa. When they arrived, you could tell they were happy they had decided to come. We spent the first two days fishing and relaxing. On the morning of the third day, my father-in-law woke up and said that his jaw was bothering him. He had just gotten a new denture for his teeth and said it was probably the initial adjustment period for it. But he was wrong. They went home that evening and he went to work the next day, where he had a massive heart attack and died within minutes. He was only sixty years old, and his death was like losing the glue that held our family together. None of us were ever the same again, and his death created a hole in my heart that has never healed. Kathy still grieves to this day.

Weeks passed, and I started to realize how much I missed working. I loved being with the kids and Kathy, but this was not reality. As always, I prayed and asked for guidance. Calls began to come in from firms, but I felt jailed because I could not work until my three months were up. I began to feel that I was losing all contact with my business clients. Although I was no longer in the office, my clients would not deal with any of my associates. Calls continued to come in and I had to tell clients that I could not work until my contract agreement had expired. The risk of losing my relationships with my accounts became very nerve-racking. Sometimes too much time to think is not good for the mind. It wanders and creates scenarios out of fear of the unknown.

After three months at home, I went back to work for a competitive firm, and it was as though I had never left. Stress and Wall Street go hand in hand, and their way of running your life is all part of the package. In 1999, I ended up working for Tradition North America. I had worked there in my earlier years, and they offered me $350,000 a year, guaranteed for three years, plus a signing bonus of $180,000 cash to join their firm. This was truly the deal of a lifetime. Most of the people who worked there were old colleagues from other firms. The best part of it all was that Tradition was now located across the street from the towers and I felt much more at ease not having to take those two elevators to the 84th floor. Even though I would still arrive at the World Trade Center by using the PATH trains below, I felt more at ease taking a short escalator ride up and down from the train platform and being able to exit to the street and arrive in a separate, safer location for work.

## Chapter Six

# *Tuesday, September 11, 2001*

September 10, 2001 is a landmark day in my mind. It is special because it is the day before my whole life changed forever. The weekend before the 11th, I had bought myself a new stereo system. It was still in the boxes the day of the 11th. I almost did not get to use it. It is amazing how we often do not have a choice in this life regarding the things that happen to us. Even years later, as I tell my story, I am still in the grasp of that day. Things have gotten somewhat better, but one week before September 11 every year, I begin to think about how I wish I could change those five hours of hell, and I am sometimes anxious and uptight before the anniversary. Looking around today, I see a beautiful blue sky and feel a warm blanket of sun just like the day the towers came crashing down along with my world.

My usual day started at 4:30 a.m. on that Tuesday morning. I was in my twenty-fourth year working on Wall Street, most of which had been spent in the towers themselves. I arrived at work at my normal time—6:00 a.m. In money markets, most of our trading was accomplished during the early morning hours because we traded with London markets and had mostly overseas exchanges. I planned to leave early that day because my wife had been experiencing severe back pain and needed me to take her to the doctor for pain shots. For several years, Kathy had been suffering from back pain, and her overuse of prescription drugs was becoming noticeable and extremely hard to live with. Meanwhile, our son Scott was starting his senior year in high school. He had always been a quiet kid, and I was worried about his future, especially his eventual transition into college. I knew he was aware of his mother's decline in health. He dealt with it by staying out with friends and, when he was home, isolating himself in his room.

But the issues at home were processed and put aside for the time being as I readied myself for what seemed like a nonstop race during the day. It was a very clear, beautiful morning. When the sun was just coming up, those towers were an awesome sight, the silver buildings reflecting the early morning sun. That morning, I met friends on the platform of the PATH train, just as I always did. As usual, we chatted briefly for a few minutes before the train arrived. It is funny, but when you have a job that entails speaking all day long, it makes one enjoy the silence. My commute was my private time. Some of us would stick our heads in the paper or chat if we had news from the previous evening. We climbed aboard the train not knowing it would bring some of us to our deaths. One friend was talking about his second child, due around Christmas. He was excited and, as usual, dressed in the Yankees jacket he frequently wore to work. I thank God we talked that morning, as it would be out last conversation. Our routine was to just go through the motions and talk just enough to stay connected before we got to work.

My friends and I spent ten or more hours a day together; more than we spent with our families. We always talked about our kids and wives and watched each other's children grow up. One good friend, Howard, had just called me the day before the 11th to chat about his son starting college. We both laughed and joked about how much it would cost for us to send them to college and how we couldn't believe we were at that point in our lives. I had watched his son grow up since he was six years old. That talk was the last one Howard and I had as he was killed the next day.

As we exited the train together, we walked up the escalator and ended the small talk. I was happy to get to work because I planned to leave early. We were all joking, saying it was going to be a slow day in the market. I can still see their faces when we stopped at the World Trade Center and the train doors opened. As we proceeded up the escalator to the lobby, I told them I would be leaving early and would see them tomorrow. We said our goodbyes when we got to the top of the escalator. It would be the last time I ever saw them. Some of them worked on the 84th floor, for Euro Brokers and the rest for Cantor Fitzgerald at the top of the North Tower.

When I walked outside the South Tower and crossed the street, heading toward Park Place, I saw the security guards who always stopped and checked delivery trucks for explosives and flammables. Although this scene brought me back to February 1993 every day, the increased security measures led me to believe we were safe from any future attacks. I got a bagel and coffee from a nice gentleman who owned a small steel cart right outside my building, as I did every day. I never learned his name, but he always called me "boss." He was located one block from the North Tower.

Work was slow that morning and, by 8:30 a.m., I started to relax, knowing I was leaving soon. My colleague Ricky and I were chatting when our building suddenly shook as if we were having an earthquake. It was 8:45 a.m. "What was that?" you could hear all over the office. I immediately jumped out of my chair, fully thinking that it was another bomb. I had already experienced that feeling, and I just knew it was not good this time. Our office was on the fourth floor of 75 Park Place, and the towers were to our right. I looked out and saw silver strips of metal like the insides of soda cans and thousands of papers falling from the sky. For an instant, it looked like the confetti that would fall on Broadway during a Yankee parade. My first words were, "They just blew up the World Trade Center!" I turned to see everyone on their telephones. I went back to my desk and received a call from my brother-in-law. He asked if I was okay. I said I was fine but that I just didn't know what was going on. "A plane hit the World Trade Center," he told me.

We had televisions throughout our office so we could watch the Money Market channel during the day. I looked up at the small box and saw the two towers, one full of smoke that was billowing like someone had just blown out a candle. There were helicopters all over the sky; they were on it immediately. I told my brother-in-law I was leaving right away. I knew from experience that if I didn't leave right away, I would never get home in time to take my wife to the doctor. This was not a good decision. If I had stayed where I was, within the confines of my office building, I would not have been witness to what came next. As I hung up the phone, my friend John was yelling that he was trying to call his brother who worked at Cantor Fitzgerald, but there was no answer. He knew the plane had gone into the tower where Cantor was located. Unfortunately, his brother never made it out. I picked up my wallet and, with much trepidation, walked toward the elevators. Not one other person was moving, just calls and calls coming in from everywhere. People were just standing and staring into those TV sets. That was the last thing I remember before leaving the office.

Everything that happened from the moment my feet touched the pavement became surreal to me. Even as I think of it today and every day, I simply cannot believe it really happened. Sometimes when I am at home and a documentary comes on television about 9/11, I will watch it just to confirm that those towers really came down. When I got outside it seemed as if everyone had disappeared. I looked up and saw a huge, gaping hole in the side of the North Tower. The street was very quiet. It almost felt like I was the only one there. I gazed back up at the tower again in disbelief, only to see the same gigantic hole that cut into the side of the building. Papers were raining down and small flames stretched out from where the plane had penetrated. I could see the defined outline of a jetliner where the aircraft had entered. There was a distinct smell of jet fuel in the air. I had no idea what was happening on the other side of the tower. I just stood there staring. I was dazed. I had no idea, looking up at the tower at that point, how many people were already dead.

I stood there for what seemed like minutes but was probably only seconds. I am sure I was in shock at that moment, but I quickly became aware of others running in panic. I was startled awake by the sound of sirens heading toward me. I decided to go left, up Park Place to West Broadway. When I reached that corner, I turned right and started walking toward the South Tower. I crossed the street because I was not able to see the North Tower from that position and I wanted to get out of the way of the people who were emerging from the buildings and coming toward me. That decision to cross the street is what saved my life that day. As I got closer to the towers, I stopped and realized people were crying. One woman was vomiting, saying, "People are jumping." *People don't jump, she must be crazy,* I thought to myself. Then I looked up at the sky again. The smoke was thicker and the flames around the tower had grown more intense. What I saw next was the most unimaginable event I have ever witnessed.

I was right on the corner of Barclay Street and West Broadway, looking up into the billowing smoke. My memory is so vivid of the first person I saw falling. I do not believe I will ever forget it. I stopped in my tracks to look up, and what I saw and felt can never be fully described in words. Through the thick cloud of smoke, a man fell head first, flapping his arms in what I imagine was an effort to decelerate his fall. He flapped in the wind, almost in slow motion, before he fell right into a restaurant umbrella in the plaza between the two towers. I had never seen a body freefall to the ground before. My body was shaking all over, and I kept saying to myself, "I didn't just see that," but the reality was that I did, and that there were more to come.

Terror is a word to describe that day. Terror is what I felt as I witnessed all of this. My mind was a camera taking pictures that would remain imprinted within me forever. I really could not believe what I was seeing. Another man: he was wearing a white shirt and dark pants. He was falling headfirst, like diving off a springboard. I pray for the soul of that man, what he must have thought jumping from 102 stories high. Those ten to fifteen seconds it took to fall must have felt like a lifetime. I can only imagine what they were thinking about on their freefall to death. Their kids, wives, significant others, or maybe what it would feel like to hit the pavement, hoping that maybe they would live if they did not hit too hard. The old tale that says that when you jump from a high place you usually die before you hit the ground is just not true. This man (and all the others that came after him), were screaming until the moment their bodies joined with the pavement. I never expected to see humans splattered all over the sidewalk and to this day, I still have nightmares of that scene. Blood everywhere, bodies lying in blood, red everywhere. I was frozen in place; I just could not move and I knew everyone around me was in shock, too. One body after another kept coming down. Some had their shirts off. I remember a man and a woman holding hands as they came down feet first. Their hands seemed cemented together, literally holding on for their lives, and I truly believe they helped each other have the courage to jump that day. I remember this woman's skirt just flapping in the air like the famous photograph of Marilyn Monroe standing over the subway grate with the breeze blowing up her dress. They were frozen, stone-like, as they waited to hit the ground. When they hit, I was so completely sick inside. I just tried to get my mind focused on what was happening, to comprehend what was going on before my eyes. People were waving their arms in vain, like baby birds learning to fly. To see people crashing into the ground is something your mind just cannot absorb or ever erase from your memory. In addition, the sound was unbearable. As each person hit the ground, it sounded as if an enormous sledgehammer had just hit metal. The sound was maddening. I thought I would go insane if it did not stop.

My mind was so overwhelmed with what I was watching unfold before me. The people on the streets were screaming, "What's happening?" Policemen and firefighters were screaming for people to get away from the buildings. To the people coming out of the World Trade Center, they were yelling, "Don't look back! Just keep moving!" There were bodies falling all around the North Tower, and you had to dodge them as you moved. The police were trying to maintain some sense of order and keep any kind of movement away from the buildings. The whole street around me was nonexistent as I was so focused on the tower and seeing these individuals, some of them probably my friends, jumping to their deaths. Mangled body parts, bodies that had arms and legs snapped, heads that were bleeding all over the street. Some of the people were burned and screaming, cut and bleeding, crying for help.

When those people hit the ground, I hoped to God that they died immediately. I often wonder whether I would have been brave enough to jump or instead burned alive at 1,700 degrees. I cannot imagine that any of my forty-six friends who worked on the 102nd floor may have had to do that very thing. Would the heat of the fire be so bad that I would not be able to take it anymore, or like all of us believed until that day, would somebody rescue us and get us out of that inferno?

While I was focused on the North Tower, the South Tower exploded above me. The heat immediately hit my face. A huge fireball and parts of the building began to rain down on everyone who was standing there watching. The second plane had come in from the opposite side of the South Tower and gone right through, as I stood there with many others. All I remember is that it was like a huge flashbulb going off in my eyes. I turned to my left and ducked quickly around the corner of a building, which initially shielded me from the pieces of the aircraft that were falling. It was a mad scramble for cover. Directly across the street, I saw a door that I thought would allow me to get into the building, but, when I reached it, I saw a sign saying it was locked due to renovation. In the door's glass reflection, I could see all the debris dropping down out of the sky, falling behind me. This was only seconds in real time. My reflection in that glass door on a dead run, trying to get in, will stay with me forever. As I grabbed the locked door handle, I thought, *This is how I am going to die.*

I closed my eyes, pushed futilely on the door and waited, sure that something would hit me. There was glass scattered about, and I could see pieces of fiery metal coming at me. The noise was deafening, there was panic and screaming, people were falling and being trampled. Again, I am sure it lasted only seconds, but it felt like minutes. I then heard people yelling, "They're blowing everything up!" I stepped back from the doorway and saw that there were bricks all over the sidewalk. They had come down from the top of the building, where pieces of the jetliner had crashed. In the pile of bricks, I saw arms and numerous other body parts. I panicked, turned and looked right at another man who was standing in the middle of the street. He was wearing a dark blue suit and holding a cell phone. Our eyes met, but we never said a word to each other, and I could see he was also shocked that we were still alive. The top of the building I was standing in front of had collapsed onto the sidewalk, and under the bricks were three people who had been standing there, now crushed. All I could see were two arms sticking out of the fallen brick with no movement at all. It was so unbelievable that nothing had hit me. The debris was everywhere. That man and I were the only survivors left on that end of the street. I will never forget focusing on him, speechless.

Once again, what seemed like minutes was only seconds. There were keyboards and pieces of computer screens strewn everywhere. As I was looking around for a place to escape, the cars on the street started to explode from the heat and flames that had sprayed down onto them. I thought it was more bombs. I began to run toward City Hall in an effort to get away from that area. I jumped over bricks, metal, and bodies, determined to find shelter or just to run. When I made it up the street, I saw City Hall. There were police officers standing on the steps with rifles ready to fire. As everyone was running around and screaming, I realized that City Hall might be next. My mind was racing all over the place and I started to panic. I didn't know where to go. Then I remembered what I had done the last time—the ferry. I knew the ferry would be running. My heart and soul kept screaming for me to get out of there. I felt that time was not on my side. To get to the ferry, I had to go back toward the towers. Everyone else was going in the opposite direction. I could now see the destruction of the second tower and still did not know it had been caused by another plane. I thought it was a bomb. People were still jumping one after another, and as I got closer, I could see in the faces of others passing me, covered with dust and some bleeding badly, the looks of shock, dismay and total fear. Explosions continued as the gas tanks of nearby cars were ignited by the balls of burning jet fuel.

I tried not to look up as I walked against the crowd that was walking uptown, away from the towers. I made my way down to the ferry platform near Moran's Bar and Grill in the Financial Center. People were starting to line up behind me as we waited for the boats to arrive. Even if you did not look up, the events people were describing as we stood in line that day were so unreal. You could hear the bodies crashing into the façade of the North Tower. It had a huge canopy outside to protect people from the elements while waiting for cabs. The banging sound was unbelievable as more and more bodies hit the roof. I have never wanted to leave a place so badly in my whole life.

I knew I had to get across that river, and it took what seemed like forever to get on the ferry. There were two boats, one for Jersey City and the other for Hoboken. My boat didn't have many people on it, just two women who sat behind me, crying and saying over and over, "Let's leave," as they watched people fall out of the smoke, other people hanging out the windows, waving shirts and ties, anything to get someone's attention. I prayed so hard to God to get me across the river. We finally pulled out, and I remember just thanking him that my life had been spared. As I looked back, I felt relieved that I was finally moving in the right direction, away from the hell that had just happened.

When the ferry pulled into Jersey City, I got off and started to walk toward 101 Hudson Street, the place where I always parked my car. I then heard what sounded like the bending of steel and loud crashing. As I turned, right before my eyes, the North Tower disappeared into a plume of white and gray smoke. As the building fell, it sounded like an avalanche. I could not believe my eyes. People all around me were screaming and crying. I knew that there were still many people trying to help at the towers, and those fire trucks and police cars and ambulances were right where that tower had just fallen. They all had to have been killed. I later found out that people were diving under cars to escape from the building as it was falling down. Another survivor I spoke to said he was with a group of people crossing the Brooklyn Bridge, and, when they saw the smoke coming at them, they thought it was a chemical bomb that would kill them once the smoke reached the bridge. I knew my friends had just been buried alive if they had not already jumped. I did not know what to think; I was full of shock and disbelief, and my heart was pounding so fast I was out of breath.

The North Tower was gone and, although I could not really see what had happened, it looked like a bomb had dropped and released all this toxic smoke. I did not know what to think at that point. I thought that I was safe but realized the building where I had once worked had come crashing down with my friends inside. Little did I know that most of them had died instantly when the second plane hit, all burned alive either at their desks or waiting on the 80th floor for the elevators to come up. I now know that everyone was told not to leave the building, that the building was secure. I knew in my heart that the people who worked for Euro Brokers had tried to leave immediately after they heard the explosion, a lesson learned from 1993. I turned away, walked toward my car, and just stood there, numb and in total disbelief at what had just transpired.

I cannot remember how long I was in the parking garage when I heard another huge rumbling similar to the first. There was a radio on at the time, and I heard it say that the second tower had just come down. All the other people in the parking garage began running over to the side to try to see out toward the World Trade Center, but I just stood there thinking the world was ending. People went absolutely out of their minds. They were screaming and holding their faces. The whole thing came down right in front of my eyes. I did not know what to say. I just stood there. I then tried to get my car out of the garage, but the parking attendants would not let me. They were afraid the garage was going to be blown up as well. No one knew who was doing what. It was utter chaos. The only thing to do was to try to get as much information as possible from the local radio station. After a long hour of waiting, we were finally allowed to get into our cars and leave.

Suddenly, I realized that no one in my family knew that I was still alive. I did not carry my cell phone all the time, but since that day I do not go anywhere without it. I took my phone out of my glove compartment and saw that there were messages but no service. It killed me not to be able to contact them. Quite honestly, I did not know if my wife could handle the state of uncertainty. I could not reach a soul and could only wait for the cars ahead of me to move down the exit ramp as I wept and tried to make some sense of what had just happened.

Exiting the garage was very difficult and the traffic was at a standstill for miles. I looked back and saw an enormous, billowing cloud of white dust, all that was left after twenty-four years of seeing a skyline that was now changed forever. I turned up the radio and the newscaster was screaming. I heard him say Washington had been hit and that we were under attack. It took more than an hour to be able to get onto a main highway. My anxieties were so high I was having trouble breathing. I made my way very slowly up to the New Jersey Turnpike and started back home the way I had always gone, except to my left was now destruction, chaos, death and the end of my world as I had known it. The terrorists had finally done what they said they were going to do: destroy the World Trade Center.

As I drove along the Pulaski Skyway, it was eerie not to see oncoming traffic heading toward New York City on what would normally have been a busy day. I saw State Troopers standing outside of their cars along the highway at the Statue of Liberty exit, clutching their rifles in anticipation while waiting for their orders. I finally reached the Turnpike, hoping it was not closed. I was able to enter and make my way toward Route 78 in New Jersey. I realized the signal for my cell phone was now working. As I picked it up, it started to ring. It was my wife. "Where are you?" she asked frantically. I was so upset and happy to hear her voice I could hardly move my lips. "I'm on my way home," I said. "I made it. I'm alive." I could not say anything else and so I just hung up. I looked to my left at the downtown skyline and saw the aftermath of what appeared to be a nuclear holocaust. Everything was changed now; my eyes were seeing a completely different world from the one I had been in at 4:30 that morning. I began to pray. My life had been spared and I made a pact with God to change my life. I was thinking I would never be able to go back, but how could I do that? I continued to drive and stared into the lane in front of me. I had driven Route 78 for eleven years and knew the road by heart. The usual fifty-minute ride took what seemed to be hours. All the way home, even with the radio on, I kept seeing those poor people jumping out of the building and hitting the ground. In fact, I still see them today. I cannot get the nightmare out of my mind.

While I was driving home, my daughter, now twenty-one, was on her way back from work. All she knew was that my brother-in-law, Joe, had spoken to me at 8:46 a.m. Marie worked with Joe at Merrill Lynch in Hopewell, New Jersey. He had called her into his office to explain that he had spoken to me and that I was leaving the building. Later, he called her back into his office after the first tower fell and told her it might be a good idea to go home. He believed I had been in the building trying to get the train out of the city when it came down. Marie and her fiancé drove home thinking there was a good chance I had been crushed when the tower fell. When they arrived home, my wife told them I was okay, and my daughter collapsed.

My son, Scott, who was in 12$^{th}$ grade, had been watching it all on TV in his classroom. My daughter went up to his school to get him and bring him home. He later told me that when they called his name out in class to go to the office, he feared the worst. He said that as he walked down the hall he could see his sister waiting for him, crying. That walk down the hallway, he later told me, was the longest distance he had ever gone in his life. But then Marie told him I was on my way home and that I had not said anything else.

When I got home, everything looked different: my house, my kids, my wife, all the trees and everything around me. I was home, in my own driveway, and I had not died. Everyone came out to meet me in the garage and I just gave in to the overwhelming shock I was feeling, weeping, crying, and trembling. My wife immediately took me to our family doctor, a man who had been not only my doctor but my neighbor for eleven years. When I described the events I had seen, I could see total shock on his face. This was a man who had delivered babies, seen many illnesses, and saved lives. Yet it was obvious that nothing had prepared him or anyone for this event. He strongly suggested that I see a therapist as soon as possible.

When we arrived home, it felt like I was at my own funeral. There were twenty-two messages on the answering machine from my sisters, my in-laws, from friends whom I had not spoken to in fifteen years. The calls continued to come in as I detailed each sequence of events that had unfolded that day. I was still checking with my wife and the television to verify that what I had witnessed had truly happened. When my sister called, her first message was calm, but by the third message, she was screaming for my wife to pick up. For a brief period, my family truly thought I was dead. I stood in my kitchen listening but not really comprehending that this is what it would have been like if I had not made it home. I felt so humbled to know that people loved me that much to call to see if I had made it out. I was listening to loving comments and thoughts that I would never have known about if I had passed. I went to sleep early that evening after taking a couple Xanax. I just wanted to escape to my own room and bed. I still did not really understand what the next days and weeks would bring. Who would? I was not able to sleep that night and, after about two hours, I went downstairs. I sat in my chair in the family room and let the feeling of safeness surround me, knowing I was in my home. It was very quiet and dark and I felt hazy from the medication. I bent down and hugged my collie, Scottie, so hard I practically choked him.

The hours rolled into morning and, in my distant consciousness, I could hear the phone ringing constantly and my wife telling everyone I had made it home. I sat there wondering how many of my friends and acquaintances had died. How many innocent people were dead? At times, I found myself jumping around in my chair as if I was still running from death. I was afraid to close my eyes because I could not bear seeing those people jumping over and over and over again. As I replayed the events in my mind, I realized I had almost made a fatal mistake by leaving my office as soon as I had. I could have walked right into the second incoming plane. My instincts to get out had been based on my experience with the first bombing in 1993. We never know what lies ahead; we just react.

I had a yearning to turn on the TV. I was devastated and yet I was craving more information. Somehow, if I got enough or the right information, I could make sense of all of this. Maybe I just wanted some validation to make sure I was not dreaming. I saw the news and the huge light they had shining down on the carcass of what had once been the World Trade Center. It was totally gone, brought down to a pile of steel girders covered in dust, which was the crushed remains of my friends and coworkers. The news said many were missing and their whereabouts were still not known. I began to shake again and reached for a Xanax to calm down. My good friend Tom's wife called and said he had contacted her around 10:00 a.m. the previous morning. He worked at Cantor Fitzgerald and had said everyone was sitting in a circle, holding hands and praying. "The floor is getting very hot and I want to say goodbye in case I don't get out. I am going to go join hands now with the rest of my colleagues who are sitting together praying. The firefighters will be here soon. I love you!" he said. With that, he hung up the phone and, soon after, the entire building collapsed. My friends freefell to their deaths. They were on the highest floor you could possibly be on and the bottom literally fell out from underneath them. I imagined that they were the first ones to drop as they sat there optimistically waiting to be saved. I am sure there was no television reception at the time, so they did not know the severity of the situation. I know they said the floor was hot, but they were able to sit in a circle and pray. I often wondered what was worse, jumping out of the buildings or burning to death. I could not imagine. I am sure it did not take long once it fell. In the end, they all fell out of the sky together, hopefully all holding hands and not alone.

I think of all the money the finance industry has generated and the many people who lived such comfortable lives. No amount of brokerage could have changed the outcome of that day. I know of two friends who were not at work on September 11th, one who called in and extended his vacation by an extra day and the other who took a sick day. More calls came in and, as the days went by, I realized many close and personal friends had died. It felt like a part of me had died as well.

These were people whom I not only had working relationships with, but also personal ones; people who had helped me learn my job and had been at my house many times. We had watched our kids grow up together and become young adults. It was just such an unbelievable amount of loss. I can remember looking out the window on the 84th floor of the South Tower, over toward the Statue of Liberty, many times when I worked for

Euro Brokers. Who could ever have imagined a jetliner entering that very floor and incinerating so many of my colleagues? Some died, I learned later, just by choosing the wrong stairway. A friend called and told me he had been notified by authorities to bring in brushes, combs, toothbrushes—anything they could use to match DNA from bone samples that were found. I had taken my shirt off when I had gotten home from the doctor, but I did not see until two days later that I had burn marks all over the back of it from the explosion at the second tower. When I saw that, I realized once again how lucky I was to be alive.

## Chapter Seven

# *Life after September 11*

The day after September 11th continued into the night, and I finally gave in to the fact that I was not going to be able to sleep again that night. My Xanax-induced calm only slowed down my physical body; my mind was still running rapidly. I kept staring at my digital alarm clock, watching each minute pass with a new thought of what was now going to be. I crept out of bed slowly so as not to wake my wife. I wanted to be alone. The night was still, as it had always been when I arose to go to work, but this time everything around me seemed different for the second day in a row. This was now my new reality. I quietly walked downstairs to greet my faithful pal, Scottie. Even he looked so different to me. "Why am I alive?" I said to myself. "How did I get home unscathed?" The downstairs clock read 4:00 a.m., and my stomach felt as though I was on a rollercoaster. I put on some coffee and noticed a red flashing light coming from the phone in the dark kitchen. I walked over to see the twenty-two messages that had been unanswered. My heart began to pound rapidly, and I wondered if I had the courage to play them. Even though I had listened to them once, I had not really comprehended what they had said. I waited for the coffee to be ready and decided to hit the playback button. I turned the volume way down and began to listen to the play-by-play of that awful morning. The first message was from my sister, Marie. "Kathy," it said, "please call and tell us that Bill is okay. Thanks." Then my sister Lynne called right after Marie, when the second plane hit. She was upset but her tone remained calm. All calls went unanswered; my wife had not been at home to receive those first messages. She had been in the waiting room at the car dealership when the service manager came running into the room to tell everyone to turn on the TV. When Kathy saw what had happened, she started screaming for them to give her the car back, saying she had to leave immediately. They tried to calm her down and told her to go home and wait to hear from me.

I sat down on my kitchen chair and continued to listen to the messages on the machine. The third message was again from my sister Marie. She was screaming for my wife to pick up or call her back. The emotion in both voices in those three messages was of panic, fear and shock. I continued to listen to the rest of the calls, and it made me feel like I was at my own funeral lying still in my coffin, silent, unable to utter a word but being able to hear the voices of my friends and loved ones and the anguish they were feeling. I sat down and just lost all train of thought listening to the many voices I had not heard in a very, very long time.

That Sunday, September 16, my boss called and told me that they had found an office to relocate to directly across the street from the Empire State Building. They were opening back up that Monday. It was a huge cafeteria-like room. I said I would see him then. I went to bed that night hoping to get a peaceful night's sleep, but my anxieties kicked in again and I panicked. There were multiple scenarios going on in my head. How would I get to work? Would I be safe there? Feelings of insecurity and vulnerability overpowered me. The night before I was to resume working, I woke up several times and found myself walking around downstairs, half asleep. My heart was pounding. I was sweating. I still was not able to process all that had occurred less than one week prior. All I kept thinking of that night was that I would have to take the PATH train to 34th Street and then switch to a subway train, which would take me to the Empire State Building, my final destination.

I did not understand what was happening inside me at all. I just could not get this feeling of uneasiness out of my mind. I saw pictures in my head of everything that had transpired on the 11th. Now I would have to find a way uptown. What would happen if they started blowing up the subways or the tunnels? When I turned around on the day of the attacks and saw the white cloud of smoke, I had told myself I would never go back. As I thought more and more about this, the memory of not only September 11th but the attack of 1993 kept coming into my head, and I finally said to myself, "There's no way I can do this. They are going to blow up the subways. I'm not getting on that train."

I could not stay still in my bed. I was sweating, walking back and forth in my room and saying to myself repeatedly, "I can't go back, I can't go back. But I'm a man and I have to support my family. What if I can't go back?" After much deliberation, I called my boss in the morning. I told him that I needed more time to regroup. It had been such a very short time before they were up and running again, and I just could not work that way. Euro Brokers and Cantor Fitzgerald were now out of the equation because Cantor was 99.9% destroyed and Euro Brokers had lost many people. That meant huge money for the companies that could operate again as soon as possible. Accounts would move to whichever company could serve their needs. There is no loyalty when it comes to trading. I knew my company would rebuild swiftly and be back trading as quickly as humanly possible. Like it or not, business and the stock market keep going through thick and thin, even death.

Within days of the attack, I began seeing a therapist. He was a trauma specialist, someone who is used to listening to other people's pain. I went to see him in the hope that he would be able to help me deal with what I had experienced. His name was Jim and, as I began to give him a detailed description of what had happened, he just sat there and stared at me with his mouth wide open. He had nothing to say to me. What could he say after I had just told him that I had seen a head splatter on the sidewalk? What can anyone say? That is what I was thinking at the time. He sat there looking at me like a deer in headlights because he could not understand; nobody could understand what was going on because the horror I had seen had not been shown on TV. They were just showing little bits and pieces very quickly. Most of the camera people got as close as they could, but they knew they had to get back; therefore, the true picture of what was going on was mostly unseen by the rest of the world.

Jim made me repeat that story three times a week for the next four or five months. He was trying to desensitize me, I guess, although I still cry when I go through each event of that day. "You need to go through it, Bill," he would tell me. "I know in the beginning it's going to be horrible for you but you have to keep on doing this." So, I would spend the first 25 to 30 minutes of each session retelling my story.

As the days went on, the calls continued to come in. I had to verify for myself the names of my dearest friends who did not make it that day. Forty-seven had died, all of them close to me from many experiences over the years. Every day since has been filled with pain and fear. My life has never been the same. I continued in therapy three days a week, which now became my full-time job. For the first six months, I couldn't stop crying as I described the events of that day to my therapist over and over and over again. But no one is ever going to be able to erase the pictures that replay in my brain. I was forever changed. I had come to realize that this was the beginning of my post-traumatic stress disorder.

A friend who had also survived the attacks called to tell me that he had returned to work on September 17th. On his way into the city, his bus had been stopped at the entrance to the Brooklyn Battery Tunnel. Everyone had to get off, and soldiers were there with dogs sniffing all around the bus. The soldiers were sticking very long rods with mirrors on the end in the undercarriage to look for bombs. He explained to me that his stress level was so high at the time he thought his head was going to explode. The following day they evacuated the Empire State Building because of a bomb scare. Every time I heard these stories, I prayed I would never have to go back to that again.

The days that followed consisted of an early rise from bed. By 10:00 a.m. I would take two Xanax and go back to sleep for at least three or four hours. When I took those pills, the pictures in my mind would temporarily fade and I would feel safe enough to fall asleep. I would wait until about 5:00 p.m., go out to the hot tub in my back yard, and drink a bottle of wine.

I stared up into the sky praying for the souls of my friends and all the other victims who died on September 11th.

Spending the weekdays at home was something I had not done in a very long time. I began to see some unbelievable things unfold before me in my very own home. It was not long before I realized that my wife was totally dependent on pain medication because of a chronic back issue. The decay of her body and mind and her inability to control her thoughts and emotions were devastating for me to observe. At that point, she was very addicted and was consuming many pills every day: Percocet, Xanax, and Oxycontin, to name a few. Although her back pain was legitimate, she was overmedicating. She was seeing several different doctors who did not know about each other and they were all writing prescriptions for her. It was painful to watch this, and I felt like my head was in a vice because I was unable to fix it.

Looking back, I should have realized that Kathy had a problem with pills in July of 1999. She had called me at work and said she was addicted and needed help. I just told her she needed to cut down the amount of pills she was taking each day and try not to rely on them so much. I hadn't wanted to face it or take the time out of my life to admit that my wife had a dependency problem. The sad thing is that when someone is hooked on that many pills, they turn into someone you do not know or even want to know anymore. From 1999 to 2001, her behavior was unbelievable. My children were very upset, as she was decaying right before their eyes. I managed to sweep it under the rug, however, because I was always too busy doing what I did best, pretending that everything was fine, and Kathy was very good at putting on a façade. Now that I was home every day, I had no choice but to acknowledge her addiction. I left my own pain and suffering on the back burner and tried to focus on her. It became so bad that she seemed as if she was in a coma daily. We were going to hospitals, doctors, and pain specialists at least three times a week. She would send me for prescription refills and I could not, or would not, think about the oddity that I was going to three different pharmacies for her. My prescription plan would cover a certain amount of pills per month, so she started seeing multiple doctors, not letting the others know that each one was feeding her addiction. I was still functioning in my own haze and I felt safe being at home, so I did what I had to do to keep my wife sedated and create as little conflict as possible.

On one occasion, I went to the pharmacy and the pharmacist told me it was too early to have the prescription refilled. I called Kathy from the car and she said, "I'll call you back. Don't leave whatever you do." I sat in the car like a robot waiting for its next command and, within minutes, my cell phone rang. "Go back in," Kathy said. "It'll be okay." Apparently, she had worked her manipulative magic and convinced the pharmacist to refill her medications. I complied; for me, it was safer to be home than to go back to the death and destruction of New York. I was not able to piece it all together at that time. I was not stable myself. With the prescription filled, my wife was content for another couple of weeks.

One day I was with my therapist in a session when he made the statement, "There's something else going on with you, Bill. What is it?" I told him my wife wasn't well, and we began talking about my situation with Kathy. I was only about two or three months into counseling at that time, and each session had focused on the events of September 11ᵗʰ, not my home life. "I need help with this, Jim," I said. "She's on drugs all the time." I desperately needed someone to step in and help. I brought Kathy in to see Jim with me two or three times. The therapist was totally pissed off at her for not acknowledging her addiction and the behavior that was preventing me from being able to work on my own losses. She continued to insist there was nothing wrong with her and that all the issues in the house were my fault. Couldn't anyone see what was happening to our family? No one, not even my therapist, gave me the help I needed to handle Kathy's progressing addiction.

In the meantime, my own dreams became more intense, imagining I was back working with my friends who were dead. In my dream, I would keep saying to them, "We need to leave the building. It is not good. It's not good." They always seemed to move so slowly in these dreams and I could not find a way to make them listen to me. It was almost as if they were frozen, trying to put one foot in front of the other. In another dream, I would be crying to my friends about how sorry I was that they had died. In one case, my friend Eric said to me, "Bill, we're okay, don't worry." That was a very vivid dream and it helped me to let him go.

Christmas was approaching, and it hurt when I thought about it. It had always been my favorite holiday with family traditions, the music, the decorations and many gatherings with family and friends. Now all I could think was, *What is it all for?* I needed to know what lay ahead. There seemed to be no direction or purpose in my life now. I did not know my place anymore. Was I supposed to work? I did not know what to do.

I was numb, I was out of my element, and I was living in a situation that was no longer in my control. My wife suggested I see a woman who was very similar to John Edwards, the psychic medium who could communicate with people who have died on the TV show "Crossing Over." I was skeptical because I do believe in God and, as a good Irish-Catholic, I knew this type of thing was frowned upon in the church. I decided to comply and made an appointment to have a one-hour session with this "spiritual connector."

When I walked into her establishment, a feeling of calm and peace came over me. Her office was filled with statues of saints, and I sensed a feeling of reverence for a higher power. I introduced myself and, as we began to speak, she knew immediately what I had been through and gave me information that was uncannily accurate about past friends and family members without my telling her anything. She truly was a very good source of strength for me. Initially, I did not realize I was going to connect with past relatives and some of my friends as well. The one that affected me the most was a man named José. He had been our guard at the front desk at Euro Brokers. I knew he had roots in the Bronx, where I was born. José spoke through this woman and told me that I had always treated him with respect and had never looked down on him. I would talk to him every morning over coffee and just ask how his family was. I had genuinely liked José. When the woman spoke, I immediately knew it was him, and I also knew right then that this woman had the ability to speak to the dead.

She told me I had many guardian angels around me, not just one, and that my aura was very strong and bright. I felt somewhat comforted by her words and began to believe that I had survived for a purpose, perhaps to write this very book about all the suffering that occurred after that tragic event. She said she was being shown the wheels in motion and that my life was on a new path, changes were coming, and I would be able to help others. Through her words, I knew my friends had made it to a better place and felt comforted that someday I would see them all again. What I did not know is that I had to go through much more personal suffering before I could get to a place where I would eventually be able to help others. I went back to see her again later, when I was debating about whether to return to New York City. I missed my job very much and did not feel good about myself. Who was I? No one knew the real me. People could only understand so much and for so long before they forget the living hell I was in every day. Flashbacks, uncertainty and total depression continued to consume me.

# Chapter Eight

## *Denial*

The loss of life and career has been a very tough pill for me to swallow. The few close friends I have left have never been the same since that tragic day. Many turned to alcohol or lost their marriages to divorce. We all had very lucrative jobs, and yet we were extremely vulnerable every day we entered those towers, subconsciously thinking we were safe from the outside. Personally, I still do not know what happened but can honestly say the word "terrorism" is truly a word with which to reckon. As my therapy continued, I started to realize what the words "post-traumatic stress" really meant. I had no feeling toward anything or anyone and often went out for long walks to speak with God and ask why such a terrible thing had happened. However, every time I thought about it, my mind became cluttered with feelings of guilt and sadness. I felt guilty that I was not happy and thankful to have survived, and I felt sad because most of my friends had not. I had never been more conflicted in my entire life than at that point.

As the daily news focused on the recovery of bodies, I soon realized there were not many to be found, just small pockets of remains. That was hard to believe because I had seen so many people fall to their deaths. What had happened to all those bodies? I fell into a deep depression, as I knew all I had worked so hard to achieve was slipping away. I still had a substantial mortgage and, as I discovered by being at home full-time, a wife who had developed a very serious drug addiction. I thought I had a perfect family compared to what I had come from; we had made it from nothing, and my wife and I truly loved each other very much. As in every home, there are always problems, but trying to work through them was proof that you really cared for one another. We had promised each other through thick and thin that we would never part and would always take care of the other. Unfortunately, when the two players became dazed on a daily basis and sought the other for help, neither was capable. It all deteriorated very quickly.

I began to focus on the immediate problem of our bills—the ones that I had never known we had accumulated. Besides our daily living expenses, there were credit card bills, four to be exact. The smallest balance was $15,000 and the highest was $26,000. Where had all this money disappeared to? On one hand, Kathy truly did take care of the household needs, but I did not understand the true extent of her spending. Prior to 9/11 she would often present me with a $100 bottle of wine when I arrived home from work. Little did I know it was a smokescreen to justify her own spending on frivolous items for herself. No matter how much I was earning, it seemed like it was never enough. Kathy would get these impulses to venture into things she knew nothing about. She always needed to be in full control of everything and everyone. During the Internet boom in 1999, she called me at work one day and said she wanted to start day-trading stocks. She had no experience in the market but it sounded good to her. I told her that she should instead get a job to take up her spare time, but she said that working around the house was her job. She then called my financial advisor and started to harass him. He called me at work and said he was not letting her do this because it would destroy all we had built to that point. Kathy continued to call and barrage both of us daily until he finally contacted me and said he no longer wanted to deal with us and terminated our relationship as clients. She had won again. All of these things would resurface during my therapy sessions later on.

What I had ignored for years was about to destroy our very existence. The house had to go. At that point, I was not sure whether Kathy was taking more and more meds to try and hide from the reality caused by years of spending way above her means, or from the fact that the cat was now out of the bag. Where were we going to get the money to pay off these balances? I was so distraught, and I continued to become more depressed

Kathy was right alongside me, regressing more and more. Going to the emergency room was like going to the store because we frequented it so often. After hours of waiting, they would give her the pills for her back pain and we would go home. Kathy was refilled once again. I would get her to bed after she had spent a whole day in a semi-coma on the couch. Finally, I got my break and I would crawl into my hot tub with a bottle of wine and two Xanax. As I sat in the tub, I would stare up into the sky and become fixated on the stars. After two or three hours of trying not to feel any emotions, I would come into the house and just pass out and go to sleep. I still could not get the picture of those people falling to the ground out of my head. It would not turn off.

During the days that followed the destruction of the towers, my daughter and son were very quiet in the way they were going about their everyday business. My son constantly retreated to his room and Marie had a full-time position at her job. She and Ryan were actively making plans for their wedding day. The best way to describe that time is that we were all functioning in a kind of semi-conscious coma, on autopilot. We were just existing in our home, listening daily to all the updated news about the attack. Scott became progressively more detached from Kathy and me. His schoolwork began to decline, and he grew afraid of how our lives were changing. He had a difficult time with me being home and with his mother's deterioration. Marie, on the other hand, worked all day and any free time was focused on planning for her wedding, an event my wife was unfortunately not well enough to help with.

None of our family members stepped in to help because we were the ones who had always helped *them* financially. My insurance policy was the first thing to be liquidated. We received a sizable check in the mail, which helped us to pay off some debt and catch up on our mortgage payments. The insurance policy had irked Kathy for ten years because the premium was withdrawn directly from my paycheck and she saw that as less money for her. Every year she tried to manipulate me into canceling it but did not succeed.

In the meantime, my employer had stopped paying my full salary. Initially I was put on a temporary leave of absence with the assumption that I would be returning to work. I was told I had to wait three months for my long-term disability insurance policy to take effect. Each month it cost $8,000 to run our household and pay the bills. In the past, this had not been an issue, but now it was nearly impossible. Kathy took over power of attorney and began to liquidate other assets as well. I was not in a right frame of mind and, even though she wasn't well her-self, I just let her have her way with the finances. It was so hard to care anymore.

Meanwhile, my dreams became more intense. I was always seeing buildings crumbling with windows blown out, standing by myself in a place where there was nothing but desolation, chaos and rubble. I would feel in my dream as if I were the only survivor after a nuclear bomb. No one was around me. I really did not want to sleep anymore. Afraid to close my eyes at night, I would fight the return of the dream until sheer exhaustion would prevail.

I had been in therapy with Jim for over a year when I finally realized that my progress with him had reached a plateau. He had gotten me through those early weeks and months reliving the tragedy week after week, session after session. We mutually agreed that he had done his job. At one point Jim said to me, "Bill, you know it's never going to change for you. I am glad you got your disability and I am glad I was able to help you do that but you do realize that you are scarred for life, don't you? All I can do is tell you the truth. You worked out some things with me and the rest is going to take time. You are going to continue to have ups and downs and I hope to God one of these days it goes away. I have never experienced anything like your story be-fore and to tell you the truth, I do not know what else I can do to help you. Terrorism in this country to the degree of September 11th is new to us as Americans and we just don't know how to handle it." *Well, that's pretty positive,* I remember thinking sarcastically to myself. I left and went home.

I soon realized I wasn't going to be mentally able, with or without medication, to deal with this on my own. As if things were not bad enough, my sister Marie called to let me know that my father was in the hospital due to liver and kidney failure. She wanted me to consider going to see him to say goodbye. As I expressed earlier, I really was not a big fan of my dad. In fact, at times I hated him. My sister and I talked for a few minutes, and I told her I would consider it and call her later. "Bill," she replied, "he really doesn't have long. Maybe two or three days at best. So if you can live with his passing and not seeing him again, so be it." I had not spoken to or seen my father in fifteen years. He had treated me extremely badly all my life, and I really did not need to add this to my plate. The 11th had given me a completely new perspective on letting go.

I brought Kathy into the conversation I was having in my mind and told her how I felt. I only had one mother and father, but I wanted to weep at the thought of going to see him. I finally decided I was going to be a bigger man and say goodbye. Was I doing this for my sister or myself? As quickly as I had decided to go, I changed my mind. Why should I have any emotional attachment to this man? My hot tub was my church, and in it I asked God for guidance and strength. I found solace in its warm waters and really worked through many of my difficult decisions there. Respect kept coming to mind—even if he had never respected me, I felt I should respect him. By the time I went to bed that night, I had decided I would go see him the next morning.

The drive there was an hour plus, but I had so many thoughts of what I would say or feel, it seemed like only minutes. I lost complete track of time as the miles passed under the car. I entered the hospital and made my way to his room. I saw my mom sitting next to his bed just staring into his face with a look I could read like a book. I saw her eyes seeing him at age twenty-six again, coming to pick her up for a date and having their whole lives ahead of them. I then focused on my sisters around the other side of the bed, staring at him and thinking of their own personal time with him as children. I realized that I had been the only missing link in the circle of chairs around the bed, as I had been for many years. I stepped forward and made the circle complete for the last time. He was coherent and I think very embarrassed for all he had done to me when I was a young man; or at least, that is how I was going to remember it. Whatever I had been seeking from my father in that visit, I did not find. No great words of wisdom or apologies came from his lips. We did not exchange many words and eventually I hugged him and asked God to bless his soul. I spent several hours at his side and left knowing I had done the right thing.

He passed away the next day. I really loved my father in my own way and thank him for the things he gave me. He chose to be cremated, which was very surprising for our Catholic upbringing. I later found out he had died with no money to pay for a funeral and had made sure none of us would do so. We respected his wishes, and we each have an Irish urn full of his ashes in our homes. He and I are finally living together again.

# Chapter Nine

## *Moving Forward*

Not long after my father's death, Kathy told me she had made me an appointment with a new therapist who dealt specifically with near-death experiences. At that time, Kathy was supposedly seeing a female therapist for her own drug issue, and the therapist's husband was in the trauma field. The thing about Kathy was that she knew how to play people. Kathy was well into her drug use by now and when she went in to see this woman, she told her an absolutely convincing story. When she was done, the woman never knew she was on drugs. She talked about how her family had fallen apart after September 11th, the pain she was suffering with her back ailment, and how her husband was a "trauma guy." The therapist then suggested that I make an appointment with her husband Larry because that was his specialty.

The first time I walked into Larry's office I was very forthright and asked him to explain what he meant by "trauma." "Well," he responded, "I've had people in here who have basically been in serious car accidents hanging upside down with the seatbelt on and gasoline dripping on their right arm knowing that the car they were trapped in was going to explode at any minute. Is that traumatic enough for you?" I told him it was close, and then asked if he wanted to hear my story.

As I began to talk about my experience with my second therapist, his reaction was similar to that of my prior therapist—sheer disbelief. Now here was a man who had heard numerous stories of gore and disaster, yet he was overwhelmed by what he was hearing from me. All he had to say was that I should come in twice a week.

Larry began using Thought Field Therapy, a technique developed in 1982 by a man named Roger Callahan, and it seemed to work for me. It was a kinesthetic approach that combined my emotions with my bodily sensations. By now, I felt like a seasoned veteran at explaining not only September 11th but what I was living with at home. Larry tried to convince me that I needed to work on one thing at a time, not realizing that I was drowning and waving my arms to be thrown a life preserver. After a brief honeymoon period with him, I started to soul cleanse. Kathy and I would compare notes after our weekly visits to our husband and wife therapists. I began to understand Kathy's twist on her daily life at home. Sadly, her perspective did not even minimally resemble what was really transpiring. I took it upon myself to ask Larry for a roundtable discussion with his wife and mine. I really felt the need to hear what my wife was saying with neutral parties in the room.

Our appointment was set and that morning was like all others. Kathy was high on pills and I was at my peak stage of post-traumatic stress. When we arrived at the office, I was seated across from Kathy's doctor, and Kathy was seated across from mine so we could see each other's eyes and facial expressions. The meeting began with Kathy's doctor telling me that, from what she had gathered from Kathy, I was an alcoholic, verbally abusive, and, for most of our marriage, selfish. Out of all that was said, I truly had been guilty of alcohol abuse at times, as well as speaking out of line. However, when I was called selfish, I exploded on everyone in the room. After thirty seconds of rapid-mouth fire, I asked the two doctors, "How do you fix drug addiction?" With that, Kathy's face dropped and her therapist froze. I proceeded to explain what had been going on for the past four years. Kathy's doctor sat up straight in her chair, glanced over at Kathy, and asked, "Is this true?" There was no response. I turned to Kathy and asked if she had told her doctor about her addiction to pills. Again, Kathy had no response. Kathy's therapist then asked me if I wanted to save our marriage. "No way," I said. With that, I got up, went out to my car, and waited for Kathy to join me. My head was pounding and I just wanted to run and hide. That therapy session was cathartic for me in that I was finally able to tell someone the truth about Kathy.

After that, I began walking three miles a day to get a break from everything. Each day, I contemplated whether I was strong enough to leave. My conclusion: not yet. But I became more emotionally detached from Kathy as each day passed. When I walked, I felt that I was seeing for the first time the trees changing color, my son going to school, seasons changing; things I had never had time to see before because of my job. It seemed so unreal to be in this situation. I was finally able to enjoy all the things I had worked for my whole life, yet I was losing them at the same time.

As I watched the money deplete and my wife's continued slow decay, my stress level continued to climb. I realize now how bad I was. I got no sleep at night and, when I did sleep, I dreamt of planes crashing, or running into buildings and waiting for them to collapse with me inside. I knew that if I did not make a change soon, we were going to lose everything. All that I had accomplished in my life was disappearing before me. I had prayed every night since I was a kid that I would not be like my dad or have to struggle like my mom, only to end up with nothing. That was all very difficult for me to accept. It was not all about the money though. It was that my marriage and my family were crumbling right in front of me, falling into an endless abyss just as the towers did on September 11th.

My wife's health was deteriorating drastically from the large amount of medication she was taking. I finally needed to call 911 one day after she had not eaten or drunk anything for several days. When the ambulance arrived at our home, they took her out on a stretcher and I remained behind to help the State Trooper finish his report. I later learned that the ambulance had to stop on the way to the hospital to perform emergency CPR on Kathy. Apparently, her heart had stopped beating and her vitals were gone. They were debating calling a medevac helicopter to take her to Morristown Hospital, which specializes in trauma, but they were able to resuscitate her and continued on to Hunterdon Medical Center instead. I did not handle the stress very well. I sat in the emergency room for five hours and became very agitated at my wife, who had caused this addiction because of her own inability to cope with what had been, prior to September 11th, a very good life.

After much research, we finally decided that Kathy should have back surgery. In 2002, she had an operation which consisted of having three discs replaced and a bar inserted into her spinal column. She was immobile for three months while I cooked and cleaned and tried not to lose my mind. As she began to improve physically, the drug dependency did not. There were a number of emergency room visits between 2001 and 2003. She also went into a drug rehabilitation center twice. The days were long and confusing. At one point, we even tried to go to therapy again as a couple to learn how to function in a world and routine we no longer knew. She fought the therapy and any attempts to help get her off the drugs. "I don't need help," was always her response. "I have a back issue."

Meanwhile, I still had not accepted or dealt with the loss of my friends, my job and almost my life. My daughter Marie had moved in with her fiancé several months earlier. They had decided to have a house built, and they asked if they could both move back in with us for a year. I was so glad to have them at home; it really helped me. When Marie saw the stress that Kathy was putting on me concerning her medication, she offered to administer Kathy's pills. My daughter felt she would be able to control them better than I could and get her mom to stop abusing the pills. Within two weeks, the pressure was so bad that Marie gave the job back to me. Kathy was relentless in her constant demands for more meds. No one was going to tell her she could not have as many as she wanted, when she wanted them. It was a nightmare living this way day after day. I called some friends and family and tried to have an intervention. Bad move. Kathy yelled and told everyone to go to hell. I stopped caring anymore and continued to separate emotionally from her. I was so tired of fighting this losing battle.

Still, we went to Kathy's pain specialist every two to three weeks. At that point, I was more of a driver than anything else because I was taking her either to doctors' offices or to hospitals all the time. This probably saved me, or at least I thought so at the time. I was so busy taking care of her that I did not have to deal with what had happened to me. The doctor asked Kathy about some meds he had given her because she was claiming they were not working. He told her to give back the remaining pills and he'd write a new prescription. She looked at me and said, "Well, I don't know what I did with them." Then the story changed to, "I never filled the prescription." Continuing, she then said, "I think I flushed them down the toilet." I sat there listening in astonishment as she changed her story three times in less than sixty seconds.

The doctor then looked at me and asked, "Bill, what is the real story?" I just sat there, not knowing what to say. The doctor got very angry with both of us and asked me if I was selling the meds he had prescribed for Kathy. I told him he was crazy for even thinking such a thing. He decided to call the pharmacy and see if we had filled the prescription. I was so angry with Kathy for putting me in such a situation I was ready to explode. I could feel my blood pressure rising with each passing moment. As soon as the doctor left the office, I started screaming at Kathy to tell me the truth. In hindsight, I now believe she had taken the pills well before the prescription should have run out. The doctor walked back in, told us that she had filled the prescription, and said that he could no longer provide her with medical care. He removed her from his patient list because he was extremely worried about losing his doctor's license as a result of Kathy's misuse of his prescriptions. I yelled at Kathy all the way home. The pressure in my head was indescribable.

Every morning after that, I had to make a choice whether to work out or start drinking. I convinced myself that drinking was not the answer. I had to be strong, and I realized that I would drink myself to death if I let go. At that point I basically did all of the cooking and cleaning in the house. In between doctor visits, my therapy, and Kathy going for pain shots in the back, the days went by very quickly. I anxiously waited until sunset each day, when all my household chores would be done and I could finally go out to my hot tub to escape my current life.

I regrouped and told myself that one of us, meaning me, had to remain sane for the sake of our son. Yes, sane. The word was nowhere near the state in which I lived. I looked at my beautiful daughter, who was getting married soon, and imagined how it must have been for both my kids to see their own parents disintegrating before their eyes. I made a decision that I had to make a drastic change. I convinced myself once again that drinking was not the answer.

## Chapter Ten

# *The End of My Marriage*

I always knew I would be paying for Marie's wedding day, and plans were made. As I scrambled to come up with the money, I realized that if I did not write a check and physically hand it to her, then we might not have any money left to pay for it. Kathy tried to argue over this, but I finally took control and withdrew the last of our savings. My kids were coming first from now on. I knew Kathy had lost all sense of right or wrong and would no longer be involved in any of my monetary decisions.

Finally, about two years after 9/11, I decided to leave my wife. I had thought about it for months. Kathy had been out of control for years. Scott had retreated to his room, his friends, and was now doing drugs on a daily basis. I felt like I was the only sane one in the bunch. But how was I going to present my decision to my family? My only source of income now was a monthly Social Security check. It was completely gut-wrenching. The whole thought of leaving made me sick, yet I knew it was something I had to do.

Marie and her fiancé, Ryan, had moved out of the house and into the home they had built together. One evening when they were over for dinner, I decided that I would tell them all as we sat down at the dining room table. Kathy was absolutely out of her mind on pills, and I said, "Look, I'm going to be moving out of here." Marie turned white as a ghost. Both she and Scott had known this was coming eventually, but they did not realize I had already made up my mind. Scott did not say a word. I knew there was an apartment available for me and Scott about three miles down the road. I could live there for a while and keep an eye on Kathy and the house.

I said to them, "This is the deal. Things are not happening the way they should anymore. I'm not very well myself and your mom's out of control." I then looked right at Kathy and continued on. "You don't listen in regard to your medication, you do what you want, and you're in a fog three-quarters of the time. Now you're obviously sick, and I know you are going to twist things around and say that I'm leaving you because you're ill." Turning back to face my children I went on. "I'm telling you all right now that is not what I'm doing. I am not doing that because I would never leave anybody who is sick. It is not in my nature. Kathy, you've known me since I was nineteen years old. I would never leave you if you were sick with cancer or anything else. You choose to do what you are doing and now we are basically bankrupt and we're losing our house." Turning back to Marie and Scott, I said, "I go downstairs to the basement every morning and by ten o'clock I ask myself whether I should pop twelve Xanax, drink two bottles of wine, or lift weights. To tell you the truth, I usually lean toward the pills. Instead of jumping on the bandwagon, I need to get out of this situation because I am the only one here that you are going to have left down the road. One of your parents has to be sane. I am very sorry but that is what I have to do."

Kathy was speechless at that point. She did not react because she was so many Oxycontins in, that her head was bobbing; but we were all used to that behavior by now. She did not even know what was going on. "I'm not saying that I am going to divorce your mother. I need to leave to get a little bit of space and figure out what I am going to do."

The next week, I left Kathy and took a two-bedroom town-house rental not far from the house. We both knew she was not capable of caring for Scott, so he decided to come with me. My disability check had come in and there was enough money for Kathy to pay the bills for the time being and for me to take care of my newly-incurred expenses. After I moved out of the house and into my new place, Kathy would call four times a day and abuse me over the telephone. After seven straight days, I could not take it any more and verbally retaliated. It was at that point that I knew the marriage was over and I was filing for divorce. Initially, Scott stayed with me because of Kathy's instability. Over time, she really put pressure on him to be with her, as she did not want to be alone. Eventually, he chose to move back in with her. He truly suffered the most from all of this. Scott had been just a carefree seventeen-year-old prior to 9/11 and then, without warning, he had to deal with two completely unstable parents. He was hurting from the pain of the breakup. All he wanted was to enjoy his senior year in high school. I just wanted to run and hide from everyone; but, for the first time, I finally felt free of all the responsibility I had been carrying.

## Chapter Eleven

# *A New Beginning*

After much discussion about the price, Kathy and I listed our house with a local real estate agent. When the "For Sale" sign was placed in the front yard, I felt very conflicted, torn between feeling happy that the huge financial responsibility of the house would be off my shoulders and sad because the place where we had built our foundation for the last thirteen years would no longer be ours. We had experienced life in that home, and I suddenly felt that I was giving up my shell of protection.

I had tried to explain to Kathy that all of our possessions, both monetary and material, would be divided evenly. I always believed that her job was as difficult as mine; in fact, it was probably much harder: cooking, cleaning and raising two children. I explained that, if she would read the terms of the divorce, they were more than fair and it would save us both money and a lot of mental stress if she would just sign the papers. At first, she agreed. But I should have guessed that she would become angrier as the divorce proceeded. I assume she did not believe I would really go through with it. The papers were delivered on her birthday without any prior knowledge of when they would arrive. That added a completely new dimension to the divorce, as I had nothing to do with the poor timing.

As I could have foretold, the only piece of information she really cared about was why I was divorcing her. I asked my attorney when I filed why I just couldn't site irreconcilable differences. But New Jersey law stated that the divorce would not be granted for that reason alone. He then asked why I was really getting divorced. I answered with two words: substance abuse. He explained that the substance abuse would have to be documented in my filing. At first, I thought about how that would look for Kathy and, even worse, my kids. The reality of seeing it in black and white might be too much for them to bear.

Scott explained later that he had witnessed Kathy's receipt of the divorce papers. He told me that when her eyes focused on the words "substance abuse," she went insane. She began swearing and screaming my name aloud, like I was the one who had gotten her involved with the drugs in the first place. Her behavior following that day was indescribable.

Filing for divorce had caused a great rift between me and my children. Even though they saw what was going on, they still did not want me to leave their mother. They also felt that I was leaving them the burden of having to care for her. The battle between Kathy and I over the divorce continued for the next year.

As this was all happening, our house sold and Kathy had to move. Although she was no longer my responsibility, I still felt obligated to make sure she and Scott had a decent place to live. He insisted on staying with her, as he was now attending Chubb Institute of Technology for computer programming. Kathy and I both received close to $100,000 after the sale, so I knew she would be okay financially for a while, but her previous spending habits were a great concern. As I predicted, the money only lasted one year. She eventually had to sell all of the furniture we had accumulated during our marriage, which she had kept through the divorce. But she was only able to sell it for one-third of what we had initially paid.

During that time, Kathy was admitted to and then checked herself out of several rehabilitation centers. Sadly, she never stayed at one facility long enough to get well. In the meantime, she rented many different places, frivolously spending money as if she had an unending flow of cash. Kathy would become homeless at various times and beg family and old friends for a place to live. My son continued to feel a sense of obligation to remain loyal to his mom.

Meanwhile, I had my first taste of being solo. I was forty-seven years old and living on my own for the first time in my life. The sad thing about it was that it did not suit me. I tried to surround myself with pictures of my kids and my old life. Many nights were spent alone just drinking wine as I stared at the pictures that had now become my only link to the past.

It was now three years since I had last worked on Wall Street, or at all for that matter. One day my good friend and ex-neighbor Chris called and asked if I would be interested in working for him. He was a very successful businessman who owned his own electrical supply company. I really was not sure what I should do. The logical answer would be to say yes. At that time, I was feeling abandoned by my family, friends and the whole world. Sitting home every day thinking about old times was not going to improve my life. How did this happen to me? I called Chris back and asked if I could try part-time work, and he agreed. I started working four hours a day in his warehouse stacking shelves. Sweating and lifting heavy boxes was now my employment situation and, believe me, I was truly grateful to him for trying to get me back to life again.

After working for about three months, I started to pay attention to my coworkers. On Friday afternoons, they would make plans for the weekend. I thought that going out and meeting some new people might be a good idea. It had been quite some time for me, and I missed being close to someone. But what would anyone think if they knew my story? That was too much to worry about. I would take it one step at a time. Meeting and speaking to people was what I had done for a living every day, and now it seemed so foreign to me. Scared, I kept putting it off. Each Monday, I would say I'd go out on Thursday night to the local pub and mingle with the crowd. I would prepare myself but, by Wednesday afternoon, I began second-guessing my decision to go. I didn't know if I wanted to be bothered getting involved with someone again. By Thursday afternoon, I had completely talked myself out of any movement toward the chance to go out. Instead, the end result was staying at home and drinking by myself while replaying old family movies on my VCR.

After a few months, I had worked my way out of the warehouse and into the office. I wanted to give my brokering skills a shot in a new industry: electric sales. Spending those months in the warehouse let me get accustomed to the components I would now try to sell for my friend's company full-time. Meanwhile, Kathy finally responded to the full terms of the divorce. On the other hand, was I finally agreeing to hers? She ended up making many demands over a one-year period, and I had finally given in to most of them. Either way, it was going to be final, and again for a moment, old memories began to play in front of my eyes.

My daughter's wedding day quickly approached. Unfortunately for Marie, her stress level was at an all-time high as a result of the divorce. Kathy, Marie, and I had all been involved in planning the wedding day from the beginning, and it was really exciting to find a place for the reception. We decided on a very exclusive golf course in Hunterdon County. As we began to figure who would attend, I knew Kathy was not aware of how many people she had severed ties with over the past few years. Many friends were no longer friends, and my family had become angry with Kathy for her consistent destructive behavior. Once I had decided to leave the house, Marie had to take full responsibility for the whole day. I was at a loss for words to describe how helpless I felt but knew I had to respect Marie's wishes, and she wanted me to leave her alone to handle the details with her soon-to-be husband.

My attendance list for the event had started off with over seventy-five people, but the reality of the day ended up with me going by myself with no family or friends in attendance. Everyone was so concerned that Kathy would not be able to keep her emotions in check and start fighting with everyone on my side of the family, and I wasn't going to take any chances on my daughter's day being ruined. The wedding was about Marie, and I wanted her day to be one she would always remember.

The day itself was beautiful, bright, and sunny, and I was so happy that I had been able to give her most of what she wanted for her special day. I truly felt the person she had chosen to be her husband was a very good man, and I felt blessed that I was alive to walk her down the aisle. When I saw Marie in her wedding gown, so many emotions came over me. I saw my little girl, now a beautiful young woman, starting her own life. I thought of how I wanted to show her off to my family and friends, and yet none of them were at the reception. But as always, God would intervene and say to me, *You're alive to see your first baby get married, so no depressed thoughts today.* It was a day that went off without a hitch, though it was not what I had pictured. But Marie will always be my beautiful daughter. To this day, she has a very strong, happy marriage, and my initial thoughts about my son-in-law were accurate. He truly is a wonderful husband and father, and I consider him to be my own son.

After the wedding, I wanted to make a clean break and I figured leaving my old town would be a good start. I headed across the river toward Bethlehem, Pennsylvania, an area I was familiar with because members of Kathy's family had lived there for years. I found a small apartment in the center of town and decided to make the move. In the process of putting down my security payment, I took a quick glance at my checking account to make sure I had sufficient funds for the check to clear. I always kept $2,500 in the account Kathy and I had originally held jointly, but I had removed her from the account when I had moved out of our house. I figured this would be a good time to use that money. When bringing up my account, however, I noticed a zero balance. My heart started racing and I tried to remember what I had done with the money. I called the bank. The branch manager informed me that my wife had written a check two days prior for the remaining balance. She had written a bad check and cashed it with our usual teller, who never checked the account status because it was a normal procedure for Kathy. Luckily, the bank replenished my account with their deepest apologies as soon as they realized Kathy's name had been removed.

I moved into my new place in Bethlehem fully aware that I was running away from everything I knew and had built since I was a young man. I put as many mementos as I could on the walls around me and, even though I wasn't in my old house, I tried to make it look that way. My job selling electrical parts was not really working out. Previous dreams of running out of buildings seemed to reappear on a nightly basis. Every time I drove on Route 78 to get to work in Parsippany, New Jersey, I would pass my old exit. Flashbacks would come instantly, remembering everything I had lost after September 11th. Xanax and wine were my two best friends, and I enjoyed more and more time with them.

## Chapter Twelve

# *Revisiting Wall Street*

In spite of now settling for a life of being alone, my relationship with Christine happened quite unintentionally. A close friend and I had set out for an evening of drinks and small talk. We decided to go to a bar that was playing a live version of the old TV show, "The Dating Game." We thought it would be fun to go and watch. We had no intentions of participating,

When we arrived, the entire back of the bar was set up exactly like the real show. It was being sponsored by a local radio station. I sat down with my friend and began to have some beers, which eventually turned into a few shots of whiskey. We watched the first round of the game and I remember thinking how much had changed from when I was young. This is how people meet each other now.

A young woman who worked for the station was walking around asking men if they would participate and she wasn't having much luck. When she approached us, I graciously bowed out and excused myself to the men's room. Meanwhile, my friend thought it would be funny to volunteer me while I was gone. Not knowing this had taken place, I heard my name called when I got back to the table. I looked around, waiting for another Bill to get up, and my buddy pointed to me. He started laughing and said he'd go up with me. Of course he didn't and I soon became the third member of the cast.

During the game, three men were asked questions by a woman hidden behind the partition. When it came to my turn, the woman asked, "If I went on a long trip for work and returned home, how would you greet me?" It took me about three seconds to respond. I blurted out, "I would put on some Sade, pour some Chardonnay, and then give you a massage." The place went nuts laughing and the radio D.J. said, "Man, I'd date you!" With that, I was chosen as the winner. When I came around and saw who had chosen me, I was pleasantly surprised to see a very beautiful woman. She had red hair and a perfect figure. We sat down together and enjoyed some small talk. Then we set a date to go out and have been dating ever since. Christine was a single parent, and I admired her strength and her optimistic personality.

Over time, I fell in love with Christine. In the beginning, it was like a breath of fresh air. She was beautiful, intelligent and we enjoyed each other's company immensely. Being with her eased my pain and suffering. All of my thoughts focused on her. I was on top of the world for the first time in two years.

Unfortunately, what I was feeling was just a break from the nightmare I had been living. In time, the nightmares came back and my euphoria quieted to a more realistic state. I then began to feel too much stress and pressure. Christine had a daughter who was extremely uncontrollable due to an undiagnosed pervasive development disorder. Had I been in a healthier frame of mind, I could have better dealt with the situation, but I soon found myself wondering what I had done. I was back in a relationship where I had no control and I didn't know what to do. Although the situation was not what I had initially perceived, I continued seeing Christine for my own selfish reasons. After dating her for six months, we moved in together and I asked her to marry me, fully ignoring everything that was going on around us. I did not know where to begin with her daughter as a parent or how to restructure a situation that was in complete disarray. However, as long as I had Christine's full attention when she came home from work each day and a partner to share a bottle or two of wine and drown my sorrows in a hot tub with, I figured that it was another day gone by that I did not have to deal with reality.

By 2005, Christine and I had been living together for some time, and an executive vice-president at Cantor Fitzgerald was considering me for a position in New York. Their company had been hit the hardest on September 11th. How ironic—it was the very place where all of my friends had died. Now, four years later, they were trying to rebuild each of their departments. They sent their people out to solicit brokers from other companies to come in and work for them. I was convinced that I was mentally okay and that I had conquered the entire situation. I began to entertain the thought of going back to work in New York. That was literally almost suicide for me. I was not sure of my purpose in life at that point. However, I knew I needed to start supporting myself again. I felt something was missing from my life. It is obvious to me now— my life was missing. Cantor Fitzgerald decided to reopen, and I considered being one of their new employees.

After a short period of negotiations, I agreed to come back. I ended up moving in with my old friend Billy, who had also survived the attacks, and we shared an apartment together in

Bedminster, New Jersey. This afforded me half the commute I would have had while living in Bethlehem, Pennsylvania with Christine and her daughter. Although my relationship with Christine had become tenuous, I continued to see her on the weekends because I cared about her very much. Even though it was stressful at times, I knew I did not want her out of my life. She had become my best friend, at the very least.

I started my job at Cantor and, as soon as I began my routine, getting up at 4:30 a.m. every day, things suddenly started to go wrong. The first morning I became really ill and upset. My instincts told me that things would never be the same and, although I was still highly regarded in my field, something inside me was missing. The circumstances were different, I was not with my family, and I had nothing driving me anymore. I was feeling like a sad, pathetic man whose livelihood had been obliterated that day in September. I felt guilty for feeling this way because, after all, I was alive, wasn't I? I should have been happy. No one was grieving because I did not make it home that day. However, I still felt that I had lost so much; my insides ached and I wanted to die. When I was not thinking of that, I did not really feel anything at all. I felt very uncomfortable in what used to be a very comfortable situation.

On my first day, I caught the PATH train to Manhattan and started to panic all over again. I got on the subway and began to curse to myself. What was I doing? My heart was racing and I felt it was not fair for me to come back. Why did I live? Why did they die? When the train pulled in, I suddenly remembered that I had promised myself that I would never, ever come back to New York City, yet there I was, walking into the very job that had almost taken my entire life not once but twice.

I continued this for one week. I kept feeling there was something not right inside, and I was just not feeling the way I did before when I was at work. Something was wrong, very wrong. Empty chairs in front of me made me think of my former coworkers who used to sit in them, the way they would laugh and complain about home life, the kids, and all the pressures of the business. I just could not process all of it. I tried to convince myself that it would all be okay. I had to get back to where I had been professionally, but I soon realized that was not going to happen. I was not capable of bringing everything and everyone back where they should be, and I simply could not adjust to this new situation. Forty-seven of my closet friends and coworkers had died on September 11th. How does one forget? How does one go on? There were too many empty chairs, and I felt that I was selling my soul again to make money. However, it was all I knew how to do, and I was good at it.

After doing this for one and a half months, I started to realize it was not going to work. There were rumors that Cantor Fitzgerald was going to merge with Euro Brokers, my former employer. I became agitated and upset trying to learn a new market, dealing with my divorce and the loss of speaking regularly to my kids. My relationship with them had become strained at best. In addition, our offices would be moving to the Euro Brokers building, which was down near the World Trade Center site. What were the chances that I would be put back into that situation? If Cantor had not merged, maybe I would have been better able to cope. Part of why I had been willing to work in New York City again was because I was working in midtown. Now I would be working right in the middle of my nightmare again. I also knew that the Euro Brokers office had put up a memorial to honor the employees who had died. The thought of having to walk past the pictures of all my deceased friends every day weighed upon me.

After one month, Cantor Fitzgerald and Euro Brokers finally announced a merger. The thought of going downtown was a nightmare for me. Everything was different. Everyone seemed new. Then one day it was slow in the office, so I decided to get up from my desk and walk over to the window just to see if it was sunny outside. I froze at that moment and realized I had not looked out the window of a building in New York City since the morning of September 11th. You hear about people going back in time in their minds, but I completely went back to that very day. I saw papers flying down and silver strips of metal and other debris raining from the sky. I had to restrain the urge to run. The reminiscent smells of jet fuel were in my nostrils so badly that I felt I could not breathe. I could not move. In the distance, I heard someone yell for me to get back to my desk because we had a new market going on. I turned and mechanically walked back, apparently as white as a ghost.

My manager noticed this, called me in the back, and asked me what was wrong. I began sobbing in front of him and started to describe the whole event that I had just experienced. He was in shock when I explained to him what I had seen. I said I could not continue working there anymore if they were going to merge and go back down to Ground Zero. He was a wonderful young man and really sympathized with me. I knew my long career as a broker on Wall Street was over. I just could not bear to do it anymore.

When I left Cantor Fitzgerald on my last day, I walked down to catch the subway back to the PATH train. I realized I was not in a state of mind to perform my job duties as I had prior to September 11th and at that point, it was no longer in my power. All of the empty chairs in my office reminded me of how much loss had taken place. I began to sweat and felt my heart pounding. When I reached my car, I decided I needed help. I drove myself to the Morristown Hospital. I needed to get some bearings on my life. I needed to separate myself from the situation and go to a place where I knew no one could bother me for a while. They accepted me into the psychiatric ward and immediately gave me a very strong sedative. I felt protected by the confines of those hospital walls and the locked doors leading to my room. I was seen by many doctors. With their help I began to realize that I was the only one in control of my emotions. I became part of a group therapy session with seven other patients.

One day when we were in the middle of a session, I started to panic. I saw what seemed to be a body dropping off the roof and passing down the outside of the window. *Oh my God!* I thought, *I'm seeing people jumping again.* I turned and looked at the doctors and was about to tell them what I was seeing when all of a sudden, I saw the scaffolding being lowered on the outside of the building carrying window washers.

My sisters and my daughter came to visit. I was really embarrassed to be in this situation. Christine came to see me often and let me know she would be there for me no matter what. That made me feel good inside. After about a week, the doctors released me and told me I would have to resume counseling. Representatives of Cantor called me regularly to see if I could come back again. When I explained what I was experiencing daily, they released me from my contract. That made me feel as though they understood what I was going through and cared about me. But I knew that I was finally finished on Wall Street forever.

## Chapter Thirteen

# *Time to Let Go*

I had not heard my son's voice in three years. He had refused to try to understand my reasons for stopping the merry-go-round I had been on with his mom. My own words were coming back to haunt me. "Always promise me," I would say to him as he was growing up, "to look after your mom if something happens to me." In turn, he had become my surrogate. I consistently called his cell once a month and left my message: "I love you and, if you need me, call me." This persistence was to let him know he could always count on me to be there for him. My calls went unanswered for over three years but my will remained strong. Kathy's family, whom I remained close with, told me that both she and Scott had packed up what belongings they had left and moved down to Virginia.

Kathy contacted an old acquaintance of ours named Paul, who had done work on our home. Paul and his wife had moved to Virginia a few years prior. She came across his name in our phone directory and began to unload her story on him. Paul, feeling quite shocked at her tale, told her that she and Scott could come stay there for a while until they got back on their feet. That is how Kathy usually made the transition from living in several places in New Jersey, then North Carolina, then Delaware, and now to Virginia. She had lost everything and had no money and nowhere to go. Kathy and Scott lived in Paul's basement with two dogs and what little remained of their belongings in boxes. Scott later told me that he would play movies on his

VCR all day and night to block his mother out. He knew it was dysfunctional but he still did not want to abandon her. Whenever she and Scott lived with someone, it was only a short matter of time before they were asked to leave. Initially, Kathy would call family members, then old friends, and lastly, acquaintances, and tell them her very believable story that she was homeless.

The end of their short stay would always be prompted by a sudden disappearance of pills from their homes, or the frustration of living with a person who was high three quarters of the day. After a few weeks, they were usually asked to find a new place to live. Now they were residing in Virginia and there was no place to go. There were no friends or family within 150 miles. No one was answering Kathy's calls anymore, and I cannot imagine what this was like for my son.

I arrived home late in the day and noticed my cell phone was ringing. I glanced at the number and my neck almost twisted off my shoulders. It was registering Scott's number. My heart began to race. I could not push the connect button fast enough. "Dad." The word went right through me. I had not heard his voice in forever, it seemed. "I have a big issue I need your help with," he told me. He then began to tell me the story. They had been asked to leave Paul's home and had no money or place to go. Kathy had contacted the 9/11 Fund and, if I called them, they would give Kathy and Scott a place to live down there for six months. My immediate thought was that this call was for monetary help again, not to talk or ask how I was or a desire to see me. Scott explained that, because I was the survivor of the event, they needed my blessing to okay the money for a townhouse. I froze in place, staring out my kitchen window and wondering if I was really hearing this. "No," I told Scott. "I've done enough for your mom. You need to come back and live with me to get your life straightened out. Your mom is on a cycle of destruction and you're on the same bike." Scott began to cry and begged me to help them. I knew that, after six months, I would be hearing from them again. But I realized that I needed to be his father, not his friend. I told him I would give them what they wanted, but that it would be my final act for them.

I immediately called the 9/11 Fund, which was now handling their case. To my surprise, the caseworker began to explain the four-page letter she had received from my son. She said she had never read anything as emotionally disturbing and heartfelt as his words, and that they had decided to advocate the funds they felt he and Kathy deserved. To this very day, I have never found out what he wrote in that mini-story of his life. I agreed to sign, called Scott back, and told him they were good to go. "Thanks Dad" were his last words before he hung up. These events drained me of all my energy. I was so upset from the conversation I immediately went to bed for the remainder of the day.

Kathy and Scott took possession of a town home and, for six months, Kathy was taken care of again, this time by the acts of my son. After that, he and I would be in contact every couple of months just to say hello. It was a start back to communicating again.

About three months after they were moved in and settled, Scott called and left me a very distressful message. "Dad, I need to get out of here. Mom is driving me crazy." He said that she was swallowing more and more pills every day, and that he had just found her lying on the kitchen floor, passed out with the dogs licking her face. There was dried vomit in her mouth. "What do I do?" he asked. I told him to call 911. Kathy needed to go to the hospital immediately. But he refused to call. "No, I'm gonna make her do it," he said. He always felt that he had to keep pushing her like a child to take responsibility. Later, he explained to me that, as he waited for her to get up, he noticed that she had not showered in days. The townhouse was filthy, and she was clearly not taking care of herself. Kathy had been a meticulous woman. She had always kept herself well dressed and groomed from the time she got up in the morning until the time she went to bed at night. For Scott to see her in that condition was devastating, and this had been going on for quite some time. She called for an ambulance when she woke up, and they admitted her immediately.

Meanwhile, I left right away to drive down to Virginia. On the drive down, I kept thinking to myself, *Virginia? What am I doing in Virginia?* I had never dreamed my life would become this. I had never imagined that I would be rescuing my son from the mother who had cared for him all of his life and now could not even take care of herself.

When I arrived at their townhouse, I could not believe my eyes. Piles of dog feces were everywhere. The refrigerator was nearly empty. There was hardly any furniture, and Kathy's clothes were in piles on the floor. They had two dogs at the time. One was the lab we had when we were together, the other was another lab she had purchased after I left. They had no money to feed them, so each month my daughter would send food for the dogs to eat. Marie had given up on having a relationship with Kathy and was not speaking to her. Scott would call when he was low on dog food and Marie would help. The backyard was covered with feces, as neither Kathy nor Scott cleaned up after the dogs. The entire place sickened me and broke my heart at the same time. At one point in our lives, we had it all: a large home, island vacations, a swimming pool and many friends. Sitting in my chair on a Friday evening and looking around my home, looking at Kathy and how beautiful she was, I would think to myself, *I have it all.* Now my son hardly had any food to eat and had not spoken to any of his friends in years.

After that incident, Scott asked me if he could come and stay with me for a while. I brought him back with me for a few weeks, but Scott still felt that pull of obligation to take care of his mom. My relationship with him had been strained at the very least. He had had to listen to Kathy's side of things, which summed up to me abandoning her. She had never admitted to having a drug problem. Scott explained to me that she had screened most of his calls, but my persistence would pave a path for him to communicate with me again.

I feel the need to explain what kind of woman Kathy was as a mother. To tell this story and not acknowledge those attributes would be very unfair to the woman whom I now refer to as "my children's mother." Kathy was a very attractive woman—beautiful in my eyes. She was always there when the children needed her. She would arrange the birthday parties, make sure our children had everything they needed, and take them to the doctor when they were sick. She kept the house stocked with food, and the kids' friends would all gather there. She was a wonderful mother until the drugs took over her life.

Kathy stayed in the hospital for about a week. She contacted Scott and told him she was going to be released. When she returned home, she began her usual routine of staying clean for a few weeks. She attained a job and, within a month, began displaying her destructive habits again. The day she got out of the hospital, Scott went back down to Virginia to be with her. It was hard for him because he wanted to go back to her and fulfill this need to take care of his mother. It was as if he had taken over my role as the husband. In March, three months after her return home, he asked if he could come live with me for a while because things had gotten so bad yet again. Of course, I said yes, and again set off in my car to retrieve him. When we arrived back in Bethlehem, he was completely crippled emotionally and socially, with a drug problem of his own. He had not had any social contact, a steady job, or any fun in many years.

Scott was extremely withdrawn and unable to function as a normal 23-year-old. He still viewed himself as a 17-year-old. His emotional growth had ceased on September 11th, as did the glue that had held our family together. He possessed an anger that had been quieted by the fact that he had to take care of his mother for so long. He was not able to think about what he had lost as the senior in high school that he was when the towers fell. His home life and his foundation had crumbled, and he was left with a mother who had taken comfort in pills and a father who had become emotionally numb.

Every time I try to maintain some sense of normalcy, something else unfolds. Whether or not Kathy would have been this bad had the towers not been hit, I do not know. I think it was all hidden and that day began her demise. She was putting on a big façade and, after I stopped working, our lives had changed; she could not keep up the charade any longer. I had no idea what was really going on behind the scenes.

# Chapter Fourteen

## *A Mad Man's Diary*

It is September 2006, and I am at my daughter and son-in-law's house. I came to her home at the Jersey Shore to housesit so she and her husband could go on vacation. It is funny because I got the chance to visit the beach today, and a memory, which I had forgotten for years, just entered my mind. I had not been to the ocean in several years and I had forgotten how it used to make me feel. As I sit back in my beach chair in the sand, I see Marie and Scott as young children. I would take them on the weekends to Avon at the Jersey Shore and let them ride their bikes up and down the boardwalk. I look around today, and my life is completely different. I feel like I have lost everything at this point. Scott only speaks to me on occasion because of his loyalty to his mother, and Marie is still in denial about what happened between her mother and me. I have a distinct hole in my heart that does not seem as if it will ever heal. My wife, my son, and my friends are no longer with me. I am having such a hard time letting go of those old pictures of my life and making room for new ones. It is a grieving process. Even though I survived, my friends and my marriage did not. I do not even have the same profession anymore. Looking out at the ocean, I remember a time when I almost drowned.

When I was in fifth grade, my mom sent me to summer camp. She was always trying to get me out of the streets. That summer I went with my other campmates to a city swimming pool for a field trip. I was nowhere near knowing how to swim because we lived in a concrete jungle and only had what we called "johnny pumps," which were turned on in the street by the local fire department so we could run through the water and stay cool, ducking and weaving around cars as they drove down the street. The city pool was marked to show how deep it was at each level. I had been jumping off the side of the four-foot part and thought it was cool to do. I met up with my friends and we started walking along the edge of the pool. One kid dared me to jump in and I did, not realizing it was eight feet deep. When I jumped in and did not feel the bottom, I began to panic and swallow water. As I tried to surface, I could see a man sitting on the edge of the pool not looking my way. I was drowning and did not know how to stop from sinking to the bottom. I was so scared inside, and trying to get my head above the water caused me to lose all control. The next thing I knew, these arms came from behind, pulled me up, and dragged me to the edge. It was my friend Jimmy. He was two years older than I and a good friend from the neighborhood. That kid saved my life. Had he not been there, I would have drowned that day for sure. I was nine years old when that happened, embarrassed, shaken up, and I just couldn't describe the way it had felt when I could not breathe and almost suffocated from the water. I know someone has always been there to keep me from harm and death. I equated that situation to how I am feeling today on the beach. Am I still drowning, waiting for someone's arms to rescue me?

Gazing out at the ocean gives me solace. I reflect on all I have gained and all I have lost. I am still alive and, at least for today, I am happy about that. This feeling constantly changes because I have not been "right" for a long time. Sometimes when

I am at home I glance over at my alarm clock, and invariably I see the numbers 9:11 and they just go right through me. What does it mean? Is it a message? Never forget? Am I supposed to be doing something in reference to September 11th?  Is it is a sign for me to reach out and help the other silent sufferers? Perhaps that is what has prompted me to tell my story. Those numbers will always be the most memorable numbers in my life. They are ingrained in my memory, and they take me back to that day I was running for my life with so many others.

Do you want to know what my definition of madness is? Madness is all those men and women who worked hard every day climbing the professional ladder only to end up as ashes. All of those people who were incinerated obviously had their remains spread over a vast amount of space below. The ashes were later taken to a rubbish dump in Staten Island as part of the millions of tons of dust and debris that were once the Twin Towers. The rest were scattered all over the people who were running when the buildings collapsed. The most sickening feeling I have from that day is realizing that people were showered not only with cement dust when those towers fell, but also with bone fragments and other human remains. All those years of work, all that education, only to end up in a pile along with years of refuse from New York City. There are no headstones, no getting up on Sunday morning to pay your respects to mom, dad, daughter or son. Their remains are lying in a place incomprehensible to you or me. Sometimes as I would drive home from work on hot summer days and pass over the Outer Bridge, I could smell the garbage reeking from that area known as the Fresh Kills Landfill.

I could not imagine those people now lying in that place. For the life of me, I still cannot grasp it. That is madness.

September 11, 2006. Five years after the day that changed me forever. I returned home the night before from staying at my daughter's house. The time is 10:03 a.m. and I have been up since 7:00 a.m. crying and emotional but not as bad as in past years. Arriving home last night, I felt a very empty feeling. I had not wanted to leave my daughter's house. I cannot help but think at 8:45 a.m. that my life changed forever five years ago today. I stare at pictures of the deceased on TV and, as their names are read aloud, I focus on the faces of the many friends and coworkers who died that day. I am empty inside but also know that I survived, and I am grateful. This trio of feelings forever plays in my mind. I pray today for all my friends and the other poor souls who passed as I almost did. I have my daughter and my son and am very grateful for a second chance, but I know that I, too, became detached that day and did not come home the same.

I notice my old boss on TV. Brian was a real gentleman. He had become a hero by helping one man survive. The wives of some of my friends got up at the podium and read the names of those who had died. One lady I saw was clutching my friend Eric's picture in her hand. I had worked with Eric for six years. We sat next to each other for ten hours a day. We both escaped from the first attack in 1993. It just breaks my heart to see their wives upset and to know that their children will never see their fathers again.

The people who jumped that day were finally shown for the first time on TV in graphic detail. I revisited in my mind the many people hitting the street and watching them desperately trying to fly. I will never be able to erase that thought, knowing some of them were people I knew more than half of my life. It is just not getting any easier to deal with. I now find it intriguing to hear other people explain what they saw from their perspectives and listening to their accounts. I can truly say my life did not flash before my eyes, however I was running for my life. I was not killed, thank God, but I died somewhat emotionally that day. Five years later, when I visit the ocean, I wish I could go back to a time when my children were small and I felt normal inside. All was well with my family and my marriage, my job, and all of my friends were still alive.

Although I am living an extremely different life than before, I am desperately trying to find peace. I am lonely but I do not always want to be with people. I tried to go back to New York but could not. I had no choice but to divorce my wife. She was spiraling downward fast and it was killing me trying to save her. I cannot explain the emptiness and all that I feel I have lost. The world goes on even when we do not. During my last days of work on Wall Street, I was earning $300,000 a year plus bonuses. Although I have lost all of it now, I did come home on September 11th and I thank God for the journey, the guts, and the energy not to quit all those years.

The days are long now and I search to find myself both mentally and, at times, spiritually. I am exhausted. The pictures of that day are impossible to erase from my memory. The people who died at Euro Brokers and Cantor Fitzgerald were friends who grew up with me through difficult times. We conquered together, watched our kids grow, and saw each other get gray hair from the stress. I miss them. I miss my job and the man I used to be. I pray for all their souls. I pray for peace for myself and for all of us.

I have finally come to realize there is nothing that can delete my memory of that day. Just as there is nothing I can do to stop all the other situations that seem to come one after another. The smallest of stresses so easily overwhelms me. The present me is someone who cannot commit to anything anymore, always aware of my surroundings and, on most days, in a complete state of loneliness and separation from all who did not experience what I did. I enjoy nothing as I did before. Music. People. Recreation. It has been five years and I wonder if I will ever get better. I really try. I think of all that has happened, but my mind wanders back on its own at different times, and I feel as if I have no control. Many pressures and traumas affected me before 9/11, but I considered myself a very strong person considering where and what I had come from.

Today, I live in a very small one-bedroom apartment. I was a Senior Vice President at one time and now I exist on a modest fixed pension because I am unable to go back to the life and location where I worked for twenty-four years. I cannot go back and visit my old offices, cannot stop anymore and have a drink after work with my buddies, no retirement party, no hugs and handshakes for a good trade. I realize that I cannot go back in time, but most days I wish for that very thing. To hold my daughter and my son when they were small, to leave for work early and feel good about what the day might bring. To not feel this knot in my stomach every day and wonder what happened, even though inside I truly know.

## Chapter Fifteen

# *The Long Journey Back*
# *My new life*

I am finally coming to grips with all that has transpired over the past eight years. My faith is strong. I know I still have holes in my heart, but things heal themselves if you let them, as long as you can find strength in what you believe in. You have to believe in something. Some of the emptiness I know is there forever, but I had to try and regain some semblance of my old life. At the same time, I do need to let go. Anger tends to overwhelm me at times and then I regroup and eventually come to realize that as more time passes, this is my new "normal." Learning to understand that post-traumatic stress disorder has become part of my regular life is a daily task. Sometimes my temper seems to get the best of me. I try to do small things around my home but it seems to be a tremendous burden to accomplish any task. I lose control only for seconds, but that is all it takes to find I have completely ruined what I am working so hard to improve.

Christine and I always made time to see each other regularly even after I had moved out. We really understood that the situations and stress we were both under had caused our breakup. We continue and try to figure out how to incorporate our pasts into one future together. But my PTSD seems to rear its ugly head without any notice. One day I was laying tile in Christine's house, for example. Having made a cut in the tile after measuring it three times, I still hadn't gotten it correct; therefore, I completely destroyed it by smashing it into pieces. I then had to regroup and look at what I had done in complete shock, asking myself why I had flipped out in the first place. If I hear a sudden loud noise, I shudder and my heart begins to pound at an extremely fast pace. I shake and it takes a minute for me to calm myself. I find these symptoms are getting worse for me all the time. I have no capability to handle any sort of stress without a lot of pain or without beginning to shake and tremble. I feel this will always be part of my life now, and I have just accepted the fact. Keeping my demons at bay is now a common practice and, when I make the decision to be an example of strength and not a victim, the satisfaction before my Ambien-induced sleep is one I am proud of. I pray that, through this story of my life, people will connect with my pattern of thinking and realize they are not alone in the way a traumatic event can affect you forever.

With much love and understanding, my family is slowly allowing themselves to get past most of what has happened. We speak to each other in a much more caring manner, and every day we realize how much we mean to each other.

The last few years for Kathy have been very difficult at best. However, she is working now and trying hard not to use pain medication. But I know that it is still a constant struggle for her. She has gotten an apartment with Scott in our old town and is trying to repair her relationship with Marie. Kathy and I see each other occasionally on the holidays. When I see her, I see all of what once was and still can't believe what we had and what is now. I thought we'd be together forever. I pray for her continued strength to fight her demons and always wish her the best in life.

I had to forgive her for all that has transpired in order to move on. Life is too short to carry so much anger and bitterness.

My daughter recently gave birth to my beautiful grand-daughter, Veronica. Again, God gave me what he had given me before, a beautiful little girl. The minute I looked into her eyes and she into mine, I saw the angels and heard, "Grandpa, you are alive to see me and hold me, and I will be looking forward to you being here for me throughout my life. I know you will have many tales to tell me. Feeling your arms around me now, I know I will always be protected and safe. Don't let me down, and continue to work on yourself for me." And with that, I truly felt I was going to make that child my number one priority. I have been pardoned from death and will never stop thanking God for that very thing. I have truly risen from the ashes.

I hope reading this book will help people understand what happened to the individuals who lived through this tragedy and what it has done to them emotionally. The everlasting mental pain and anguish are overwhelming, brought on by pictures that replay over and over in our minds as we think about that sad and tragic day.

In my life today, I frequently hear everyone say I need to find a new job and get involved in other things. It is just difficult mentally for me to deal with, to make that much of a commit-ment. I finally had to look and see where I was in my life. I have a nice relationship with Christine, and we continue to move forward. I decided to share my story because I am ready to break out of my mental asylum, get on with my life, and try to reach others afflicted by this disaster or any other trauma, who may share the same difficulties. I am finally beginning to realize that what I initially thought was a life I had to settle for could blossom into a completely new chapter in a book.

LaVergne, TN USA
08 July 2010
188872LV00002B/18/P